THE
MEDICAL
ADVOCATE

Steven E. Greer, MD

"Impressive. Well done. This is an important book.

You could be the most impactful investigative journalist, as well as investor and innovator."

Peter Pronovost, MD, PhD
University Hospitals, Cleveland
Chair of Quality Committee for the HHS
Former Professor, Johns Hopkins
Former Chief Medical Officer, UnitedHealthcare
MacArthur Genius Award winner as pioneer of hospital safety checklists

For all Americans forced to cope with the costly and confusing maze of the American medical system

Table of Contents

The Cover

The cover is a parody of the iconic 1891 portrait by Sir Luke Fildes called *The Doctor*. It depicts an old-fashioned doctor making house calls, acting as a true primary care family doctor. I added my face to it. Since this is the type of medical care that no longer exists, which our medical advocacy service tries to replace, I thought this would be a fitting cover image.

Note that the two parents are the best medical advocates. The doctor is communicating with them directly. These are some of the most important components of good medical care.

"Hello? Hello? Hello? Is there anybody in there? Just nod if you can hear me. Is there anyone at home?

Come on now, I hear you're feeling down.

Well I can ease your pain, Get you on your feet again

Relax, I'll need some information first. Just the basic facts. Can you show me where it hurts?

Just a little pinprick.

There'll be no more (pain) ahhhhhh

But you may feel a little sick.

Can you stand up?"

Roger Waters
Comfortably Numb
The Wall
1979

Foreword

This book has been 20-years in the making, literally. I hope that is why you find it to be coherent, interesting, and enjoyable to read. I have been piecing it together ever since medical school. Then, in residency I learned a little bit more about how American healthcare works. But it was not until I became a financial analyst and journalist in the healthcare space that I really became enlightened, around 2005.

Many people have encouraged me over the years to write this book, but the timing was not ripe. However, after my experiences recently with the hospital care of both of my parents, it finally felt like the right time to do this.

The term "medical advocate" is not new. It has been an abstract phrase tossed around by academic doctors for a long time. But turning it into a real service available to patients is a new concept that I created in 2019 after personal experiences with my parents and various hospitalizations.

My family of five siblings and two parents has been fortunate to dodge major illnesses. We are a fairly athletic and healthy family of Northern European descent. But my parents are getting into their 80's and encountering normal problems seen with age.

Out of nowhere, it seemed, I was getting one call after the other from siblings informing me that either my mother or father had been hospitalized. First, my father developed a life-threatening gastrointestinal (GI) bleed caused by aspirin he was taking for knee pain. That occupied us before Christmas. Then, he had a bizarre accident involving an explosion. Shortly after that, my mother suffered a rupture of a small benign tumor in her pituitary gland at the base of the brain. The "pituitary apoplexy" led to excruciating pain for about a week requiring in-patient neurosurgery monitoring.

Fortunately, they both recovered fully. But their outcomes could have been much worse had they not been lucky enough to have had a medical doctor as a son. Once I got involved, I saw dramatic changes in how the hospital staff treated my parents.

With my mother, I was not alerted until approximately 24-hours after she had been hospitalized at one of the best hospitals in Ohio, under the care of the smartest doctors. But when I arrived at her hospital room, I found her slumped toward the foot of the bed in messy sheets. It was a bed sore waiting to happen. I went to the nurses' station, and they had no idea who was the doctor in charge. The name of the doctor on the door was incorrect.

Later in the day, as two nurses and I were getting my mother situated properly in bed, a young woman walked his. She was the "case manager" and interrupted our clinical efforts. She crassly began to talk about discharge dates. She wanted to rush my mother's departure despite she being very early in the course of a pituitary apoplexy. I politely told her that we would speak later. She belligerently insisted on talking. I then told her to leave the room immediately.

Later, I went outside and made some calls. I knew how to reach the CEO of the hospital and neurosurgery chairman. I emailed them.

I then received a call from the neurosurgery chairman. He was very nice, apologized for things, and gave me his personal cell phone number. The case manager never showed her face again. My mother could have stayed for a month if she wanted to.

She left a few days later and made a full recovery at my brother's house. My brother and sister-in-law acted as a rehab hospital for a few days, essentially. It was a big help.

With my father's GI bleed, I was not alerted for several days. Only when the red blood cell counts continued to dip did my family call me in desperation.

Unlike my mother's case, he was in a small rural Ohio hospital in a shared room. His primary care doctor was nowhere to be found because primary care doctors no longer visit patients in the hospital. A new breed of doctor called the "hospitalist" has been created. They are glorified residents who punch the clock, leave the hospital, and supposedly pass off the care to the next shift. But things fall between the cracks.

My father's doctor on the day I arrived was a Russian immigrant. He was nice, but not a GI doctor, which is the type of doctor experienced with slow GI bleeds. This hospital was so small that they had no GI doctors.

I took over the care and prepared him to be transferred to a larger hospital. Then, we realized that one of the blood draws was performed in error and resulted in falsely low blood counts. Once we realized that he was stable, my father was able to leave the hospital. But not before another rude "case manager" woman walked in and presented by father, who was still extremely disoriented from hemorrhagic shock, with complex legal releases to sign.

Had I not gotten involved, and had the ongoing bleeding been a real problem, the hospitalist was prepared to do nothing. He was Nero fiddling as Rome burned. There were no plans to transfer my father to a bigger hospital. They would have likely transfused him, watched him bleed some more, and then watched him die. They would have gone home without any consequences because, after all, people die in hospitals all the time.

A couple of months after these medical emergencies, I was driving south through Georgia. When I entered into Florida, it hit me. I came up with the idea to create the medical advocacy service. I told various people and I received tremendous support.

I am uniquely qualified to be a medical advocate because I have also been a Wall Street analyst and portfolio manager investing in the healthcare sectors. I know where the scams lie. I know which drugs work and which ones are overpriced rip-offs. I know which surgical procedures work and which ones are overperformed moneymakers. I know the tricks hospitals play to make money. I also have tremendous experience with law and litigating at the highest levels of federal court. Then of course, that is all in addition to my surgical training at famous (or infamous?) hospitals, such as Bellevue Hospital in New York and Jackson Memorial Hospital in Miami.

When I now walk into a hospital and interact with medical colleagues, I see myself in them. That was me before I had the life experiences that I do now.

Doctors live in a hospital bubble where strange things happen. Bad doctors get paid regardless of their performance or patient outcomes and are treated just like the good doctors. They can kill people with accidents and not be arrested. All the while, the bad ones have huge egos because they are blissfully isolated and ignorant of the real world.

The media refuses to portray real medicine and this dark side. Society still holds doctors in high regard.

Charities raise millions for hospitals who have CEO's making $10 Million in salary.

It is that crazy system in which sick people, usually elderly and at their most vulnerable, often without any family members by their side, find themselves thrown into as they develop an unexpected illness. The difference in care given to a patient who is a relative of a doctor or has a strong support structure is night and day from those less fortunate. In far too many cases, sick and elderly are nothing but piggy banks to be raided by the "case managers"

In this book, I will explain in more detail why you need a medical advocate. The American healthcare system is the most expensive in the world because tests and procedures are overperformed. Fee-for-service will be explained. It is the root cause. Then, the lack of accountability allows for frequent and repeated medical errors.

Patients need a nurse who is on their side, sitting in their room throughout the day. They need second opinions and an independent doctor to ask the specialists why they are doing things. Also, after leaving the hospital, more and more, the patient needs help fighting back against medical billing scams.

This is what I will explain in *The Medical Advocate*. Feel free to contact us.

Quality of Life Clinic
Info@QOLclinic.com
(212) 945-7252

Chapter 1. Why American Healthcare is the Costliest and Still Not the Best

I am proud to be a medical doctor in America. The profession is still represented by honest, hard-working, highly intelligent, men and women, for the most part. Many nurses do god's work.

Most doctors have the best interest of the patient at the top of their priorities. But far too many do not, or cannot. Hospitals often pressure doctors to do certain unethical things in order to turn a profit.

The American medical system can harm the patient. This is partly due to incompetence that is rewarded by the third-party payers. It is also due to greed.

This is why all patients can benefit from an independent medical advocate. This is why I created the service.

American healthcare, any way that you slice it, is by far the costliest in the world. Therefore, one would assume that we get the most effective and safe care. But we do not. Why is that?

There are several main reasons. First is the fee-for-service reimbursement model unique to our system. Healthcare providers are paid based on the things that they do to the patient, regardless of outcome or necessity.

What if your car mechanic were paid by a fee-for-service model? They would perform unnecessary repairs that might actually harm the car. That is what doctors and hospitals do. In most cases, those fancy imaging studies, such as CT-scans, are ordered purely because they make a lot of money, while harming the patient with cancer-causing radiation. Most knee, shoulder, and spine surgeries are unnecessary. In cancer clinics and hospitals, most of the ultra-expensive chemotherapy drugs are futile and a waste of time, but the doctors earn a markup on the cost of those drugs.

The second reason the American healthcare system is costly and dangerous is the third-party-payer insurance system that creates a disconnect between the consumer (i.e. the patient) and the provider. Patients do not have the same incentives to shop around for healthcare as they do for other purchases since insurance is footing the bill (although, modern insurance has huge deductibles, and patients are starting to shop more, or use urgent care centers rather than costly ERs). Therefore, the doctors, drug companies, insurance companies, and hospitals can hike prices with impunity.

The third reason is that the providers make it nearly impossible to shop around because they keep the costs of care secret. The actual bills are disconnected from the real underlying costs. More and more, hospitals are resorting to scams that send surprise bills of many thousands of dollars to patients who thought they had in-network insurance.

Regarding the harm that is far too often done to the patient, that has been tolerated by the American healthcare system because the reimbursement systems have no real way of rewarding quality care while punishing bad providers. The best and worst hospitals in a given region get paid the same by Medicare, Medicaid, or private insurance, no matter what (and the problem is much worse for military veterans using the VA). By some estimates, a serious medical error occurs to 40% of patients. The payers have tried various programs to reward quality, but the providers quickly rig the system.

There is no real political will to change American healthcare because hospitals are the largest employers in most congressional districts. The other healthcare sectors, such as pharmaceuticals and insurance, are also powerful. Congress is corrupted, resulting in harm to Americans (which is not new, as will explained more later).

Anyone reading this is likely a tax payer. This book will now detail how expensive and wasteful is the American healthcare system. It starts by showing just how massive are the expenditures. Then, it explains the history of events that have led us all into this current mess.

The next few pages are a bit "inside baseball" or "wonky". If you are in need of medical care right now, feel free to skip over them.

National Healthcare Expenditure

The National Healthcare Expenditure (NHE) is a number tracked and calculated by the Centers for Medicare and Medicaid Services (CMS). They create a good annual report that is quite easily read. CMS oversees the largest division of the federal government with a budget exceeding that of the military.

The most recent NHE shows that the American healthcare system costs a whopping $3.6 Trillion. That NHE includes government-funded healthcare, such as Medicare and Medicaid, as well and private health insurance and out-of-pocket payments.

Of that NHE, $1.5 Billion is from government-funded healthcare. By comparison, the entire 2019 budget of the U.S. military (i.e. the four branches of Army, Navy,

Marines, and Air Force) is only $686 Billion, according to the Defense Budget Overview.[1]

At $3.6 Trillion, American healthcare comprises more than 18% of the Gross Domestic Product (GDP), making it the largest component. That is unsustainable. Healthcare is just a service industry. It needs other manufacturing industries to support it. The tail is now wagging the dog.

In the world of finance and Wall Street, when a large a large financial number grows, it is usually measured in basis points, which are just a one-hundredth of a percent. That is how yields on bonds and so forth are measured, and those objects are only in the exponent range of billions. The human brain cannot comprehend what a billion means. One trillion dollars is an even more inconceivably large number.

For something that is $3.6 Trillion in size to be growing, not by basis points, but rather by whole percentage points, is unprecedented. It is untenable. It will bust the federal budget within a matter of a few years.

The current American healthcare system is set to implode. Like a dying star forming a black hole, this event will suck in the rest of the economy and cause a major depression. Given that the housing market caused the Great Financial collapse of 2008, this healthcare event could trigger the most severe depression ever.

The biggest employer in the country is healthcare. More than 16-million people worked in the sector in 2018,

---

[1]Secretary of Defense Budget Overview. February 13, 2018
https://comptroller.defense.gov/Portals/45/Documents/defbudget/fy201
9/FY2019_Budget_Request_Overview_Book.pdf

which is 11% of the total employment. Retail is second at 15-million.[2]

Healthcare Bills are the #1 Cause of Personal Bankruptcies

Politicians, mostly Democrats, in favor of changing to a socialized medical system (also known by the euphemisms of single-payer and Medicare-for-all) like to claim that medical bills are the leading cause of personal bankruptcies. Opponents supporting the *status quo*, mostly funded by the healthcare industries, disagree. Where does the truth lie?

The debate seems to have started with a 2005 publication in Health Affairs by Harvard researchers David Himmelstein, M.D. and Elizabeth Warren (now a U.S. senator and presidential candidate). They concluded:

> "In 2001, 1.458 million American families filed for bankruptcy. To investigate medical contributors to bankruptcy, we surveyed 1,771 personal bankruptcy filers in five federal courts and subsequently completed in-depth interviews with 931 of them. About half cited medical causes, which indicates that 1.9-2.2 million Americans (filers plus dependents) experienced medical bankruptcy. Among those whose illnesses led to bankruptcy, out-of-pocket costs averaged

---

[2] Website for Bureau of labor Statistics-employment projections as of September, 2019 https://www.bls.gov/emp/tables/employment-by-major-industry-sector.htm

$11,854 since the start of illness; 75.7 percent had insurance at the onset of illness. Medical debtors were 42 percent more likely than other debtors to experience lapses in coverage. Even middle-class insured families often fall prey to financial catastrophe when sick."

According to a blog called Politifact[3], they investigated these claims:

"In a 2005 paper,[4] Warren, along with David Himmelstein, then at Harvard Medical School, found that that 28.3 percent of bankruptcies were attributed to illness or injury alone based on 2001 data. But that number grew to 46.2 percent when researchers asked about additional factors such as unpaid medical bills, lost income due to illness, or the mortgage of a home to pay medical bills. The researchers interviewed about 900 people who had filed for bankruptcy and examined bankruptcy records.

They updated their research in a paper in 2009[5] and found for 62 percent of people,

---

[3] Sherman A. "Is health care the top reason for bankruptcies, as a Florida GOP leader said?" *PolitiFact.* January 31, 2019

[4] Himmelstein DU, Warren E, et al. "Illness and injury as contributors to bankruptcy." *Health Aff (Millwood).* 2005 Jan-Jun;Suppl Web Exclusives:W5-63-W5-73.

[5] Himmelstein DU, Warren E, et al. "Medical bankruptcy in the United States, 2007: results of a national study." *Am. J. Med.* 2009 Aug;122(8):741-6. 2009.

illness or medical bills contributed to their bankruptcy. Researchers designated bankruptcies as medical based on debtors' stated reasons for filing, income loss due to illness, and the magnitude of their medical debts."

The Harvard papers created quite a stir among the hospital lobbyists, causing them to fund junk science rebuttals. Politifact goes on to state:

"David Dranove and Michael Millenson at the Kellogg School of Management at Northwestern analyzed the data and concluded that there was a causal link in only 17 percent of personal bankruptcies.

"It is insufficient to show that medical problems are associated with bankruptcy; one must also determine whether, and to what extent, medical spending causes bankruptcies," they wrote in 2006.

Himmelstein and Warren pushed back, noting that an industry group supported the research by Dranove and Millenson.

A group of economists from the University of Southern California, MIT and the Kellogg School wrote an article published in 2018 in the New England Journal of Medicine, "Myth and Measurement: The case of medical bankruptcies."

Using data on California adults from 2003 to 2007, they found that hospitalizations caused only 4 percent of personal bankruptcies among adults. The researchers acknowledged this didn't cover all potential bankruptcies from illnesses or injuries that did not lead to hospitalization, or from hospitalizations of children or senior citizens.

In an interview with PolitiFact, Himmelstein zeroed in on those caveats, saying that it led to a big underestimate in bankruptcies."

Assuming that the low-ball estimates from the hospital-funded "researchers" are correct, which they are not, then still millions of insured middle-class Americans had to file for bankruptcy. Clearly, anyone reading this book should be concerned about medical bills, even if you think that you are insured.

Healthcare Bills are Arbitrary and Disconnected from Real Costs

Despite having good health insurance and using a healthcare facility that is in one's insurance network, more and more, patients are getting sticker shock from huge surprise medical bills. The scam is this: If a doctor or other form of healthcare provider (many ER providers are not MD's these days) is out "out-of-network", they are allowed to charge any amount they wish. Emergency room doctors often float from one hospital ER to the next. They are gaming the system and billing at out-of-network rates.

These surprise bills can be many thousands of dollars for a simple ER procedure, such as a laceration or blood test. Kaiser Health News reported that nearly approximately 20% of patients received an "out-of-network" or other form of surprise bill.[6]

Horror stories include one of a young woman who received a $17,850 bill for a urine test.[7] In Long Island, a man was told that he needed emergency spine surgery (which was incorrect advice and so often given for spine conditions, as I will discuss in detail later). They operated the next day. Then, his insurance denied payment claiming it was unnecessary surgery. The hospital sent the man numerous arbitrary bills totally $650,000, forcing him into bankruptcy.[8]

Normal "in-network" hospital bills are also disconnected from reality. They are arbitrary and do not reflect real costs at all. In actuality, hospitals negotiate prices, in secret, with insurers who pay a small amount for each claim. However, if the same patient were to have no insurance, then the inflated bill would be exponentially greater. For example, the total amount that a hospital might collect for a complex coronary stent procedure would be $10,000. But if some unfortunate uninsured person suffered a heart attack and needed an emergency stent, then the bill could easily be $100,000.

---

[6] Bluth R. "1 In 6 Insured Hospital Patients Get A Surprise Bill For Out-Of-Network Care" *Kaiser Health News* website. June 20, 2019. https://khn.org/news/1-in-6-insured-hospital-patients-get-a-surprise-bill-for-out-of-network-care/

[7] Rovner J. "Surprise! Fixing Out-Of-Network Bills Means Someone Must Pay" *Kaiser Health News* website. May 9, 2019. https://khn.org/news/surprise-fixing-out-of-network-bills-means-someone-must-pay/

[8] Werner A, et al. "Back surgery saved him from paralysis. Then the bills arrived: over $650,000" *CBS News*. September 23, 2019. https://www.cbsnews.com/news/back-surgery-saved-him-from-paralysis-then-the-bills-arrived-over-650000/

As the cost of healthcare skyrockets, the burden is being shifted to the patient. From 2010 to 2015, the out-of-pocket costs for people with traditional employer-based insurance increased 52%.[9] Obamacare, which was passed into law in 2010, directly caused this.

That's right. The ACA law was nothing but a boondoggle for the *status quo* insurance company industry. I said it.

All of those 26-million or so newly-insured low-income people under the expanded Medicaid plans are paid for now, in part, by the pocketbooks of traditionally-insured patients. The overall cost outlays from the insurance companies are growing too fast, causing the companies to issue what are essentially fake insurance policies. The out-of-pocket deductible costs, and surprise billing scams caused by insurance company denials, are so great that they effectively close off access to healthcare just as if the patients were not insured at all.

If the insurance companies did not play these games, then their insurance premiums would be too high for their customers, which are mostly large companies buying plans for their employees. In 2018, employers and patients absorbed 7% year-over-year increases in healthcare costs.[10] This is untenable.

---

[9] "Aon Hewitt Analysis Shows Upward Trend in U.S. Health Care Cost Increases" *Aon Hewitt*. November 13, 2014. https://ir.aon.com/about-aon/investor-relations/investor-news/news-release-details/2014/Aon-Hewitt-Analysis-Shows-Upward-Trend-in-US-Health-Care-Cost-Increases/default.aspx

[10] "Aon: 2018 may bring highest healthcare cost hikes for employers in 3 years" *Aon Hewitt*. August 24, 2017. https://www.hrdive.com/news/aon-2018-may-bring-highest-healthcare-cost-hikes-for-employers-in-3-years/503396/

President Trump recently signed in June of 2019 the *Executive Order on Improving Price and Quality Transparency in American Healthcare to Put Patients First* that requires the Secretary of Health and Human Services to generate reports and proposed new rules that will allow patients to shop for elective healthcare services knowing the real prices charges.[11] Plans to eliminate surprise out-of-network billing are also part of the executive order. Those actions are due by January, 2020.

The Best Hospitals in the Country are Losing Money. Why?

In the course of working on this book, I discovered a 2017 Forbes article[12] that explains why the largest medical centers are losing money despite increasing revenues. The article is based on a Harvard Business School review.[13] This is something that I have been telling hospital executives for years based on my own observations. It is remarkable how similar their conclusions are to mine.

The articles conclude, essentially, that hospitals are losing money due to bureaucratic incompetence. Hospitals

---

[11] President Donald Trump. "Executive Order on Improving Price and Quality Transparency in American Healthcare to Put Patients First." *The White House* website. June 24, 2019.
https://www.whitehouse.gov/presidential-actions/executive-order-improving-price-quality-transparency-american-healthcare-put-patients-first/
[12] Pearl R. "Why Major Hospitals Are Losing Money By The Millions." *Forbes*. Nov 7, 2017.
[13] Goldsmith J. "How U.S. Hospitals and Health Systems Can Reverse Their Sliding Financial Performance." *Harvard Bus. Rev.* October 5, 2017.

are pseudo-government agencies that cannot reform themselves any better than the U.S. Post Office can.

Over decades, the wrong mission of hospitals has been rewarded by money. They are reimbursed for care on a fee-for-service model regardless of patient outcome or financial efficiency. In fact, the bigger and more complex the care has been, the more the system has rewarded it.

The true objective of a medical center is to grow expenses by increasing numbers of employees. That has been the source of their power. Medical centers are the largest employers in many regions giving them tremendous political clout.

Unlike true private-sector businesses, the real motivating force with medical centers is not efficiency and growth of the bottom-line (i.e. net-income). Instead, the goal is to grow the top-line (i.e. revenue) in order to pay for the bloated expenses. Medical centers, like government entities, are expanding tumors growing at the expense of the host with no sustainable endgame.

The Forbes article states, "Most hospital leaders acknowledge the need to course correct, but very few have been able to deliver care that's significantly more efficient or cost-effective than before. Instead, hospitals in most communities have focused on reducing and eliminating competition. As a result, a recent study[14] found that 90% of large U.S. cities were "highly concentrated for hospitals," allowing those that remain to increase their market power and prices."

Before I came across those articles, I had thought that I had been the only source to point out that large hospitals are laying off employees, from the MD ranks to the operations staff, despite the booming economy and

---

[14] Fulton B. "Health Care Market Concentration Trends In The United States: Evidence And Policy Responses" *Health Affairs*. Vol. 36, No. 9. September, 2017.

record-low unemployment. I have personally seen it with several major medical centers all over the country, such as New York University (NYU), the Ohio State University (OSU), UCLA, Miami Health, and MedStar. Hospitals listed in the articles as losing money are the best of the best: MD Anderson, Brigham and other "Partners" hospitals, The Cleveland Clinic, etc.

The Forbes article states:

> "Brigham & Women's Hospital (BWH) is the second-largest research hospital in the nation, with over $640 million in funding. Its storied history dates back more than a century. But after a difficult FY 2016, BWH offered retirement buyouts to 1,600 employees, nearly 10% of its workforce.
> Three factors contributed to the need for layoffs: (1) reduced reimbursements from payers, including the Massachusetts government, which limits annual growth in healthcare spending to 3.6%, a number that will drop to 3.1% next year, (2) high capital costs, both for new buildings and for the hospital's electronic health record (EHR) system, and (3) high labor expenses among its largely unionized workforce."

This is another trend that I have pointed out. All of these medical centers listed above are building multi-billion-dollar new hospitals and getting into huge debt. Every place I know has done this. All of them are also secretly reducing head count.

I told people many years ago that Stephen Gabbe, MD, the head of the Ohio State University medical campus, was a fool to be building new heart hospitals. I knew that demand for coronary cath-lab procedures was on the decline. He eventually got ousted, but his replacements are doing the same thing, with another huge hospital under construction.

Electronic Medical Records (EMR or EHR) are another problem. Obamacare required them to be phased in, but they have been a disaster. Inputting the text into a computer sitting by the patient is cumbersome. It slows down the caretaking process tremendously. Patients are upset that the doctor stares at a computer rather than them. Some smart doctors now hire transcriptionists to follow them into rooms and type for them.

The Forbes article goes on to state, "Digital records are proven to improve patient outcomes, but they also slow down doctors and nurses. According to the annual Deloitte Survey of US Physicians,[15] 7 out of 10 physicians report that EHRs reduce productivity, thereby raising costs."

Also, "Although nearly every hospital talks about becoming leaner and more efficient, few are fulfilling that vision. Given the opportunity to start over, our nation would build fewer hospitals, eliminate the redundancy of high-priced machines, and consolidate operating volume to achieve superior quality and lower costs."

I am repeating now what I have been telling hospital CEO's for more than a year: Hospital executives are in for a serious shock soon. The game is over. If major changes do not occur after 2020, I will be surprised.

Not only have CMS and private insurers stopped increasing rates to match healthcare inflation, but totally new forms of healthcare are arising. Efficient cash-pay urgent care centers are replacing the long-waits at hospital

---

[15] "Deloitte 2016 Survey of US Physicians. Findings on health information technology and electronic health records" *Deloitte.* https://www2.deloitte.com/content/dam/Deloitte/us/Documents/life-sciences-health-care/us-lshc-physician-survey-hit-factsheet.pdf

ERs. Soon, those lucrative surgeries that keep hospitals afloat will be performed in doctor-owned facilities.[16]

To survive, hospitals will start scamming the system. For example, they are now labeling routine admissions as "ICU" care to get better payments. New hospitals under construction have rooms that can be converted into ICUs when needed. "Out-of-network" surprise bills have been another scam recently addressed by President Trump.[17]

Meanwhile, every hospital CEO still makes at least $1 Million (and up to $10 Million) in salary running so-called "non-profit-hospitals".[18] The number of bloated "Deans" at academic medical centers grows.

To compare inefficient hospitals to the U.S. Post Office leaves out something important. Medical centers are funded by third-party-payers with no capped budget. At least the Post Office has to meet a budget. But hospitals get paid no matter what. This is why the total healthcare expenditures exceed $3.6 Trillion, is growing at 6%, and comprises 18% of the U.S. economy.

As these pseudo-government hospital chains become forced to either cut costs and shed the middle-management fat, or find new ways to raise revenue, they have turned to ultra-aggressive bill collection tactics (because downsizing is never an option for a tumor-like, ever-growing, bureaucracy). The Washington Post[19] and

---

[16] Greer SE. "Major disruption coming to hospitals in 2020." *The Healthcare Channel*. https://thehcc.tv August 2, 2019.

[17] Greer SE. "President Trump talks about plans to make hospital pricing transparent." *The Healthcare Channel*. https://thehcc.tv July 10, 2019.

[18] Greer SE. ""Non-profit" hospital CEOs make well more than $10 million a year" *The Healthcare Channel*. https://thehcc.tv July 28, 2019.

[19] Hancock J, Lucas E. "'UVA has ruined us': Health system sues thousands of patients, seizing paychecks and putting liens on homes." *Wash. Post*. September 13, 2019.

others have reported that innocent people, who did nothing wrong other than become sick, are being destroyed in the court system. Homes are confiscated. Paychecks are seized. This is exacerbating the problem of bankruptcies caused by healthcare bills.

I predict that the next big financial collapse will be triggered by the demise of medical centers and a surge in unemployment. That, in turn, could trigger a student-debt bubble, and another housing bubble, all to burst.

The $3.6 Trillion healthcare economy is fueled by printed money from the Federal Reserve. It is a false economy, just as the national housing debt was not backed by real assets (i.e. in the form of repackaged mortgages called CDO's). When false American economies implode, they have a domino effect on the rest of the world.

Of course, this scary scenario is the precise reasoning that the hospital lobbyists use anytime federal cuts or reforms are proposed. The downside to changing the *status quo* is a powerful deterrent to reform. The bigger they are, the harder the rest of us fall, and they know it. It emboldens them with hubris. Every hospital CEO reading this book will shrug it off and collect a large paycheck.

However, the day of reckoning has come. The truth cannot be quashed forever. American healthcare had a good 100-year run. But all good things must come to an end.

Chapter 2. A Brief History of the American Healthcare System

The United States of America currently is a hybrid of "socialized" and private healthcare. The Health and Human Services (HHS) runs the Centers for Medicare and Medicaid Services (CMS), which are also known as "single-payer" systems because the government is the only reimbursement agency (although most Medicare patients also have private insurance supplemental to Medicare). Medicaid, co-funded by the states, is meant for low-income Americans. All citizens, however, become eligible for Medicare after the age of 65, or younger if they have a disability.

The Affordable Care Act (ACA), also known as Obamacare, simply expanded those eligible for Medicaid. It left the private health insurance markets to continue *status quo*, with certain new regulations requiring that plans now must cover pre-existing medical conditions, for example. Nothing changed under Obamacare other than that it gave a windfall to private insurance companies.

President Trump has made it his mission to dismantle the ACA. It is all but dead now, with the Supreme Court set to rule on its constitutionality. For what remains of Obamacare, people under the age of 65 and above the income level to qualify for Medicaid can now either purchase health insurance policies through the newly created ACA exchanges or receive insurance from their employer.

This all seems normal to Americans because we have known no other way. But it is actually a strange system compared to the rest of the world.

Step back and ponder this, if you will: Why do employers control the vital life-and-death matter of our healthcare? Why are Americans living in fear of losing their jobs because they would then lose healthcare for their families? Why does private insurance even exist? Who benefits from the *status quo*?

How Your Employer Became the Controller of Your Healthcare

Prior to the Great Depression in the 1930s, Americans mostly paid from their own wallets for healthcare. The doctor would make house calls and leave a bill. People who could not afford it usually received free healthcare. Doctors truly were noble people doing god's work at the time.

During the depression, people were starving in the Dust Bowl waiting in soup lines. They could not afford food, much less doctor bills. The rise of unions allowed for some healthcare clinics to begin at the workplace, but there was a dire unmet clinical need for most Americans.

Enter Franklin Delano Roosevelt. He began expanding socialist programs in order to buy votes, essentially. His *New Deal* failed to end the Great Depression, so he created Social Security next. The American Medical Association opposed socializing medicine, and healthcare was dropped from the plan. In the meantime, private healthcare insurance began in the form of Blue Cross and Blue Shield plans, but they were purchased by the individuals, not the employers.

Then came post-World-War-II and inflation. Germany and other European nations were ravaged by inflation. To stifle it in the United Sates, caps on wages were instituted. But the economy was booming and labor was in short supply. Therefore, in order to compete for workers, employers figured out a clever way to increase income in the form of healthcare insurance benefits.

From the 1950's onward, labor unions grew and employer benefits got larger. This new third-party-payer model created the same healthcare cost inflation that we see today. It was pricing out the elderly and poor from health insurance.

Lyndon B. Johnson took over the Oval Office in 1963 after the assassination of John F. Kennedy. To help his election chances in 1964, he too expanded socialist programs. In 1965, Medicare and Medicaid become law. It is now under the agency of the Centers for Medicare and Medicaid Services (CMS).

After LBJ created Medicare, which reimbursed healthcare providers on a fee-for-service model just like private insurance, healthcare inflation drove costs up and up. Large portions of the nation became uninsured. From Nixon to the Clintons, and then Obama, various Democrats have tried to enact some form of "Medicare-for-All" plan, and they have all failed spectacularly.

The *status quo* has been too well defended by those profiting from it. One person's healthcare fraud and waste is another person's livelihood. The main employer and gross domestic product of many states, such as Florida, is healthcare. Former Florida governor, now U.S. senator, Rick Scott made his wealth on a business model of Medicare fraud.[20,21] His hospital company, HCA, was slapped on the wrist with a fine and no one went to jail.

---

[20] Sherman A, et al. "Rick Scott 'oversaw the largest Medicare fraud' in U.S. history, Florida Democratic Party says" *PolitiFact*. March 3, 2014.

[21] Schultz R. "Gov. Rick Scott took responsibility? No, he took $300 million" *The Sun-Sentinel*. October 2, 2018.

Meanwhile, even the biggest corporations in the world cannot afford the healthcare benefit costs. JPMorgan, Amazon, and Warren Buffet have teamed up to quietly build their own in-house healthcare system.

Smaller companies are resorting to limiting employers' hours so as to label them "part-time" and avoid paying for healthcare benefits that are mandated by Obamacare. The expanded private insurance under the ACA is now essentially fake insurance given that the deductibles are several thousand dollars, even after the expensive premiums are paid, making it unusable.

At the same time, the publicly-traded health insurance companies are making record profits for shareholders and paying executives huge salaries. Those companies, in turn, fund powerful lobbying efforts that control congress and the mainstream media (Have you ever wondered why you have not seen any of this on TV? Most of the TV news ads are paid for by the drug companies.)

The American healthcare model of employers footing the bill for private insurance is broken. Total spending of $3.6 Trillion, growing at 6%, is untenable, as previously discussed. Whether a politician like Bernie Sanders succeeds at creating a single-payer alternative or not, the current system will implode very soon.

Amidst this healthcare inflation that constitutes 18% of the gross domestic product, one would think that hospitals are sitting pretty. But most hospitals are financially struggling. They are resorting to revenue-generating schemes that come at the expense of quality healthcare, as I have mentioned.

Patients without a strong medical advocate on their side are often taken advantage of like a piggy bank to raid. Hospital administrators see dollar signs when a frail elderly patient is admitted. Your lonely ill grandmother spells "cha ching" for the hospitals.

Chapter 3. Innovation Made Possible by the American Healthcare System

Before I proceed to expose all of the flaws in the American healthcare system, I must point out that the world owes the U.S. a great debt. Americans were responsible for the majority of the modern clinical technology being used today. All of the new drugs are driven by the profit incentives from our country.

Prior to the 19th Century, Europeans were the pioneers. Italian Leonardo da Vinci and Belgian Andreas Vesalius are credited with pioneering anatomy and physiology in the early 1500s. English doctor Edward Jenner is credited as the pioneer of vaccinations with the smallpox virus in 1796. Frenchman Louis Pasteur discovered microscopic germs in 1861. German physicist Wilhelm Conrad Röntgen invented the X-ray in 1895, and Scotsman Alexander Fleming's discovered penicillin in 1928. But American doctors took those inventions to the next level, and pioneered the rest, for the most part.

Anesthesia, which made widespread use of surgery possible, was invented by dentist William T. G. Morton. In 1842, he used ether gas at the Massachusetts General Hospital as a surgeon removed a jaw tumor. Georgia surgeon Crawford Williamson Long was also using ether at the same time, but did not publish his work fast enough to get the recognition.

In the early 1900's, modern surgery was established at New York's Bellevue Hospital (where I trained), and then at the new Johns Hopkins hospital, by William Halsted, MD. He started the use of rubber gloves and antiseptic procedures (He was also a bad cocaine and heroin addict, which is why he moved to Baltimore.).

Before that, doctors put their bare hands inside the belly and wondered why infection killed the patients.

After World War II, numerous American surgeons pioneered modern heart-bypass open-heart surgery. They began with congenital defects and went on to replace bad valves and clogged coronaries. Vascular surgery of the aorta and leg vessels also developed at this time.

Harvard's Joseph Murray, a plastic surgeon, performed the first organ transplant, a kidney, in 1954. Since then, every organ other than the brain and spinal cord has been transplanted. Heart, lung, bowel, hand, arm, and even the face/scalp are being transplanted.

Bacterial infections were addressed by penicillin, but viral infections went untreated until the 1960's when antiviral medications were invented. Pioneering female New Yorker Gertrude Elion, head of research for what is now known as GlaxoSmithKline (formerly Wellcome), and her employee, Howard Schaeffer, started the early work on antivirals. The first clinical drug was acyclovir. Elion went on to win the Nobel Prize for developing the anti-HIV/AIDS drug azisothymidine (AZT).

In 1955, the first polio vaccine became widely used. It was invented by New Yorker Jonas Salk.

Stem cell therapy is an American invention going back to 1957 when Seattle researcher E. Donnall Thomas attempted the first bone marrow stem cell transplant. More recently, stem cells have been used to heal damaged solid organs, such as the spinal cord and heart.

Immunotherapy is the latest American invention. Starting with antibody drugs, and now human white blood cells genetically modified to attack cancer, immunotherapy is the most promising treatment for cancer.

Chapter 4. Shameful History of American Healthcare

The American medical system has a checkered past. While it is true that most of the innovations in modern medicine have sprung from our free-market system, it is also true that numerous atrocities have stained the medical profession, eroding trust. For every polio vaccine or heart transplant procedure invented, millions of other patients have also been harmed or killed. The same profit-motivating factors driving the innovation have also led to greed and corruption of government oversight agencies.

The goal of this book and our medical advocacy services is to reduce bad outcomes. Most patients still enter and leave a hospital without too bad of an experience. But far too many do not.

This book must dwell on the negatives of the American healthcare system in order to prevent future atrocities. Let's begin by looking back over the last 100-years.

Unethical Medical Experiments

The German Nazis committed horrific crimes against humanity. Their evil extended into the medical realm with doctors conducting extremely cruel experiments on live humans.

But they were not alone. Similar experiments have been conducted on U.S. soil. Ethical guidelines that we take for granted now did not exist as recently as 1950.

In the 1940's, when the nation was at war and extreme actions were tolerated, such as internment camps for Americans of Japanese heritage, so too were the ethical guidelines on medical experimenting nonexistent. Several government-funded studies harmed groups of patients by infecting mentally ill or prisoners with hepatitis, influenza, malaria, gonorrhea, and syphilis. Our own active soldiers were guinea pigs for a variety of radiation and chemical tests.

Even after the war, the egregious clinical trials on humans continued. "When the prosecution of Nazi doctors in 1947 led to the "Nuremberg Code", a set of international rules to protect human test subjects. Many U.S. doctors essentially ignored them, arguing that they applied only to Nazi atrocities — not to American medicine.

The first came to light in 1963. Researchers injected cancer cells into 19 elderly and debilitated patients at a Jewish Chronic Disease Hospital in the New York borough of Brooklyn to see if their bodies would reject them.

By the early 1970's, even experiments involving prisoners were considered scandalous. In widely covered congressional hearings in 1973, pharmaceutical industry officials acknowledged they were using prisoners for testing because they were cheaper than chimpanzees.

Holmesburg Prison in Philadelphia made extensive use of inmates for medical experiments. Some of the victims are still around to talk about it. Edward "Yusef" Anthony, featured in a book about the studies, says he agreed to have a layer of skin peeled off his back, which was coated with searing chemicals to test a drug. He did that for money to buy cigarettes in prison."[22,23]

---

[22] Stobbe M. "Ugly Past of U.S. Human Experiments Uncovered." *Associated Press and NBC News*. February 27, 2011.

[23] List of Medical Ethics cases. *Wikipedia.org*.
http://www.nbcnews.com/id/41811750/ns/health-health_care/t/ugly-past-us-human-experiments-uncovered/#.XUDLyIIspCh8

A recently published book details how our own CIA used prisoners for extensive psychological torture in a quest for mind control. [24] The "Poisoner in Chief" was a chemist named Sidney Gottlieb who was recruited in 1951 by soon-to-be CIA director Allen Dulles. Together, they used American prisoners and foreign "black sites" to conduct torture experiments that would have made the Nazi monsters envious.

For example, the now-infamous Boston mafia leader Whitey Bulger was a victim. While in prison, he was given daily doses of LSD for 15-months to determine the limits of the brain before insanity ensued. Electrocution was another tool used to achieve the brainwashing that the CIA thought the Russians had already perfected.

After the U.S. instituted stricter ethical guidelines for human studies, the pharmaceutical industry simply went overseas to Africa and other poor regions to conduct their unethical trials. This all took place just two-decades ago, and probably is still taking place.

---

[24] Kinzer S. "Poisoner in Chief: Sidney Gottlieb and the CIA Search for Mind Control" (Henry Holt) 2019

Euthanasia

A dirty secret about American medicine is that euthanasia of frail and elderly takes place daily. Doctors routinely administer large doses of morphine to end life.

In many cases, the patients are not terminally ill or suffering. They simply have been given the Do Not Resuscitate, or DNR, status. This happens in every hospital in America.

In New Orleans' Memorial Medical Center, during the worst of the flooding caused by Hurricane Katrina in 2005, thousands of patients were evacuated by manually carrying them down flights of stairs. But on the 11th floor was a nursing home leasing space from the hospital. A doctor made the decision to inject approximately two-dozen patients, that we know of, with deadly drugs to "prevent them from suffering", she argued. It was pure euthanasia. Worse, it was a poor decision because the patients would have lived through the crisis. The doctor and other nurses panicked.

However, during the criminal prosecution, a grand jury did not indict the doctor. But the outcomes of grand juries are preordained according to the wishes of prosecutors. Clearly, the medical profession had enough clout in corrupt New Orleans to get away with murder.

Big Tobacco

The story of how Big Tobacco made a fortune knowingly selling deadly addictive cigarettes mirrors ongoing scandals with the opioid pain-pill epidemic. The companies knew what they were doing and got away with it because they controlled the media though advertising spend.

Our government and American healthcare system should have protected us from this mass murder, but the FDA, congress, and doctors looked the other way. Money from tobacco lobbyists was more important than protecting Americans for those bureaucrats. The same lobbyist/oversight relationships exist today and enables Big Pharma to sell ineffective and unsafe drugs.

Psychiatric Drugs

I will explain more in subsequent chapters how the psychiatry profession and drug industry have teamed up to create fake diseases in order to treat them with harmful drugs. It is truly scandalous and classically American.

Antidepressants do not help with depression. They actually increase it. Yet millions of Americans are on them anyway. ADHD is a completely bogus disease, and millions of kids are taking the same amphetamines that were banned in the 1960's.

People diagnosed and treated for these disorders become addicted to the pills. Their brains are permanently altered. The causes of the depression are ignored and people commit suicide. Kids falsely labeled with ADHD become addicts for life.

Harmful Food

Unhealthy food is likely the biggest health problem in America, right up there with substance abuse (i.e. tobacco, alcohol, marijuana, and other addictive drugs). Bad food causes obesity, which leads to diabetes, cancer, dementia, autoimmune diseases, and many other ailments. At least 10% of Americans have diabetes, killing hundreds of thousands a year.

The number of cancers caused by dangerous chemicals in food, such as acrylamide, is hard to quantify. But few doctors would disagree that what we eat often kills us.

Every doctor has known this for more than 100-years. Yet the medical societies do very little about it. In many cases, Big Food has actually formed partnerships with the medical societies.

Sugar

I recommend to my patients and colleagues that they read the book by Robert Lustig, MD called *Fat Chance*.[25] Someone filmed his medical school lectures to University of California at San Francisco students and posted it online. It went viral and he became one of the leaders in awakening America to the perils of sugar.

The major change in the American diet that has led to the obesity epidemic has been the introduction of high-fructose corn syrup as an alternative to cane sugar. It happened in the 1970s and the number of obese Americans started to rise with its use.

High-fructose corn syrup was cheaper than cane sugar and became an ingredient in all sorts of foods that you would not expect to have sugar in them. French fries and hamburger buns, for examples, have sugar in them. It is hard to eat any processed food and not ingest sugar.

The amount of table sugar in one 12-ounce can of Coke or Pepsi is about 40 grams, which is close to 10-teaspoons of sugar. That is more than a candy bar. It is disgusting and Americans chugged this stuff for decades thinking it was the American way.

---

[25] Lustig R. "Fat Chance" Avery. 2013.

The Big Food industry realized that sugar not only made their processed packaged foods tastier, but it also made the customers constantly hungry. Sugar causes a spike in insulin, which triggers other hormones, such as ghrelin, and the person eating it is hungry a short time later. Obese patients are in a vicious positive-feedback loop: The more they eat, the hungrier they get.

Our USDA, FDA, and doctors should have warned Americans about sugar. Instead, breakfast cereals, for examples, loaded with sugar, were endorsed by the government.

You have undoubtedly seen those silly USDA food pyramids that have breads and cereals at the base, representing the largest portion of the ideal diet. It is all a crock. It is not based on science. The Big Food lobbyists made those pyramids.[26]

The easiest thing anyone can do to become dramatically healthier is to cut back on processed foods that contain sugar. If you have to open a package to eat it, don't eat it.

Antibiotics and Hormones in Meat and Dairy

Our USDA and FDA have also failed Americans badly with the safety of our meat supply. Corporate farmers are allowed to run animal factories where the cows, pigs, and chickens are made bigger by antibiotics and testosterone. Dairy cows are given estrogen to increase milk production.

---

[26] Jacoby R, et al. "The FDA's phony nutrition science: How Big Food and Agriculture trumps real science -- and why the government allows it" *Salon*. April 12, 2015.

There is no doubt that these hormones make their way into the meat and dairy we consume. Meanwhile, children in America are reaching puberty sooner, which stunts their growth, among other problems.[27]

Therefore, one would think that the possible causation link of these dietary hormones to early-puberty would be intensely studied by the National Institutes of Health or CDC. But, of course, none of our government oversight agencies seem too eager to expose such a link.

There is no need to eat dairy for calcium or Vitamin-D. I recommend avoiding daily consumption of milk. If you like the flavor of cheese, butter, or ice cream, as I do, then consume them in moderation.

Trans-Fats

Another reason to avoid processed foods is the trans-fats in them. Trans-unsaturated fatty acids, or trans fatty acids, are best known in the forms of Crisco and margarine. In salty snacks, like potato chips, they extend the shelf life and preserve texture.

Trans-fats are the main reason so many Americans have clogged arteries. These fats in the blood stream are absorbed in the blood vessel walls, turning the vessels into tubes of Crisco.

Again, it is so easy to avoid this garbage. If it is in a package, then don't eat it.

---

[27] Euling SY, et al. "Examination of US puberty-timing data from 1940 to 1994 for secular trends: panel findings." *Pediatrics*. 2008 Feb;121 Suppl 3:S172-91.

Our USDA and FDA failed us here too. Big Food runs congress and the executive branch. It is as simple as that. Agencies created to protect us are now harming us.

If I were the president, I would undertake a reform of the entire food industry, starting with these corrupted oversight bodies. No employee of the USDA or FDA, for examples, would be allowed to take a revolving-door job with the industries they oversee for five-years after leaving their government posts. I would ban all lobbyists from entering any of the FDA buildings.

Chapter 5. Fake Diseases

American medicine has pioneered most of the great achievements, from vaccines to heart surgery. This machine is so good that it is now inventing diseases out of thin air. Many diseases that cast a wide net over large portions of the population are purely manmade and bogus, designed to create more patients for Big Pharma drugs. How American is that?

OK. You might start thinking that I am a conspiracy theory nut. I wish I were. You need to understand first just how thoroughly the drug and device industries have infiltrated the medical societies.

Medical Guidelines

Any new medical "guideline" issued from some academic ivory tower of "thought leaders" comes from a formal "society", "association", or "college", such as the American Heart Association (AHA), American College of Cardiology (ACC), American Society of Clinical Oncology (ASCO), or the American Psychiatry Association (APA). These, in turn, cause the even higher-brow elitists at the National Academies of Science, formerly the Institute of Medicine, or the World Health Organization (WHO), to follow suit.

Ultimately, this industry-funded process aims to win approval by the federal government for reimbursement. The Centers for Disease Control (CDC), The Food and Drug Administration (FDA), The Agency for Healthcare Research and Quality (AHRQ), and other agencies are the targets.

The ultimate prize for Big Pharma is to get the largest division of the entire government, the Centers for

Medicare and Medicaid Services (CMS), to sign off and grant reimbursement for a particular new disease therapy. This pot of gold at the end of the rainbow comes after industry-funded junk science makes its way into industry-sponsored medical journals, which then lead to the official industry-funded guidelines from the medical societies, which finally then leads to the arrival of the gravy train (i.e. CMS and private insurance reimbursement).

As a Wall Street analyst covering the data on new drugs and devices, I am more aware of this sausage making than other regular medical doctors. I have been to most of the major medical meetings. I see how they operate. I know the "thought leader" doctors in charge and their extreme financial conflicts of interest.

But even wise and cynical I did not fully appreciate just how much the industries pulled the puppet strings on the doctors and societies until after the global financial collapse of 2008. I had just created The Healthcare Channel and was attending a cardiology meeting in D.C. However, the convention hall was a ghost town. Only a fraction of the doctors I was accustomed to at an event like that were there. I had never seen anything like it.

Why? The depression caused massive industry budget cuts and the money spicket was turned off. All of these annual meetings are funded by the drug and device companies. Walk through the convention halls and you are bombarded with advertisements. However, after 2008, those large Big Pharma banners 30-feet high went away.

Because most of the doctors at the meetings get sent there as a form of kickback by the drug and device industries, and the money had dried up, the doctors stopped going after 2008. Those medical meetings are usually in nice cities that serve as free vacations. Do you think a doctor would spend $2,000 of their own money on travel to attend a boring medical meeting? Heck no. There is no educational value to the meetings whatsoever. All of the research presented has been pre-released long before the meetings.

Fake Cardiology Diseases

"Heart disease" is perhaps the broadest brushstroke label in medicine (psychiatric labels might be bigger). The cardiologists and drug companies make tens of billions of dollars per year from medications that do nothing to treat these ailments. One reason is that the drugs are ineffective. Another reason is that the diseases are completely arbitrary and clinically meaningless. It is hard to cure something that does not exist.

Hypertension or High Blood Pressure

You are certainly confused as to what level of blood pressure is considered to be "healthy" or is the dreaded "hypertension" I know this because so are medical doctors. The guidelines are arbitrary and bogus.

Being labeled with "hypertension" is a stigma for life. It changes your health insurance applications. It forces you to take costly medications with side-effects. It makes you a walking annuity for the cardiologist and drug company.

The hypertension threshold of blood pressure was lowered in 2017 from 140 mm Hg systolic over 90 mm Hg diastolic (i.e. 140/90) to 130/80. But the scientific evidence to support these changes was lacking. There have been no large clinical trials to support these guidelines.

An essay in The New England Journal of Medicine by George L. Bakris, MD and Matthew Sorrentino, MD stated[28]:

> "Ultimately, although the guidelines expand on [the 2003 guideline by the Seventh Joint National Committee] in useful ways, it is problematic to shift the threshold for hypertension to 130/80 mm Hg...
>
> By reclassifying people formerly considered to have prehypertension as having hypertension, the guideline creates a new level of disease affecting people previously deemed healthy. According to this definition, about 46% of U.S. adults have hypertension, as compared with about 32% under the previous definition.
>
> ...there is concern that a new disease designation can become a mandate for pharmacologic treatment without consideration of the patient's risk level. ... the guideline recommends daily sodium intake of less than 1500 mg — a goal that's difficult for many people to achieve and that was derived from short-term studies in which diets were controlled but minimal outcome data were collected.
>
> Though reducing sodium intake is desirable for people with hypertension, the data supporting daily intake of 2300 to 2400 mg are very robust, and further

---

[28] Bakris G, et al. "Redefining Hypertension — Assessing the New Blood-Pressure Guidelines." *N Engl J Med* 2018; 378:497-499

reduction has minimal additional effect on blood pressure

Another concern is the 10% 10-year-risk designation, which is not based on randomized, controlled trials;

… Although we appreciate this concept, a one-size-fits-all blood-pressure goal is problematic.

Although the new guideline lowers the blood-pressure goal for people over 65, it suggests that 30-year-olds and 80-year-olds should have the same goal. Achieving that goal is impossible for many people, especially those with poor vascular compliance (i.e., pulse pressures above 80 to 90 mm Hg), who typically have dizziness and poor mentation as their systolic blood pressure approaches 140 mm Hg."

Conveniently for the drug companies, these new drug-funded hypertension guidelines also recommend dropping the cheap and effective generic beta-blockers, such as propranolol, from the first-line therapy. They want you to use their much more expensive branded drugs.

The essay concluded with:

"Ultimately, although the guidelines expand on JNC7 in useful ways, it is problematic to shift the threshold for hypertension to 130/80 mm Hg. Some people with blood pressures of 130 to 139/80 to 89 mm Hg who are at higher cardiovascular risk may benefit from earlier intervention, but though such a broad-brush approach may be fine from a public health perspective, it could overburden our primary care physician workforce. Proper blood-pressure measurement is critical but time consuming. The unintended consequence may be that many people, now labeled as patients with hypertension, receive pharmacologic therapy that's unlikely to provide benefit given their low absolute risk, and they may therefore experience unnecessary adverse events."

Metabolic Syndrome and Pre-Diabetes

There is a good chance that some doctor has told you in person or on TV that you might have metabolic syndrome or pre-diabetes. What the heck are they? These diseases did not exist when I was in medical school only 20-years ago.

"Metabolic syndrome is a cluster of conditions that synergistically increase the risk of cardiovascular disease, type 2 diabetes, and premature mortality. The components are abdominal obesity, impaired glucose metabolism, dyslipidemia, and hypertension. Prediabetes, which is a combination of excess body fat and insulin resistance, is considered an underlying etiology of metabolic syndrome."[29]

Why was this clever medical euphemism for obesity created? First, it sounds more like a "disease" that is scarier to patients than obesity does. This is called "medicalizing" something. It gives the white-coated doctor more authority

---

[29] Mayans L. "Metabolic Syndrome: Insulin Resistance and Prediabetes" *FP Essent*. 2015 Aug;435:11-6.

to inform you that you have "metabolic syndrome" than it does to tell you that you are fat and need to go to the gym.

Secondly, metabolic syndrome beautifully combines all of the indications for cardiology drugs into one mysterious diagnosis. "Impaired glucose metabolism", which is not even diabetes, can now be treated by these costly fancy new drugs you see on TV ads. Non-diabetics are now being prescribed diabetes drugs, such as thiazolidinediones, GLP-1 agonists, and DPP-4 inhibitors.

Those are the generic terms and unfamiliar to you. Perhaps you have heard of instead Trulicity, Byetta, and Victoza, which are GLP-1 agonists. Perhaps you are more familiar with Januvia and Onglyza, which are DPP-4 inhibitors. The TV ads bombard you.

But these new drugs, which are the real reason we have "metabolic syndrome" as a new diagnosis, are not selling as well as expected. They are ineffective and unsafe. They do very little to cure diabetes but do cause serious adverse events, such as debilitating joint pain and pancreatitis.

In my medical practice, I often take patients off of medications like these. Also, statins are the other class of drug overprescribed.

Hypercholesterolemia

Pfizer's drug Lipitor was the biggest blockbuster drug in history. They really manipulated the cardiology community beautifully. It was a masterful exploitation of the American healthcare system.

As I will explain more below, cholesterol-lowering statins, such as Lipitor, do nothing to reduce the risk or stroke or heart attack in the majority of people taking them. In most cases, hyperlipidemia or high cholesterol is overdiagnosed and over-treated. People with elevated lipids should simply cut out the bad food in their diets.

For those people who have significantly high lipids, or familial hypercholesterolemia, the statins achieve nothing for them either. New classes of antibody drugs do work well, but the drug companies priced them so high that insurance companies will not allow them to be used in most cases.

Fake Psychiatric Diseases

Psychiatry is the perfect specialty for Big Pharma to dream up fake diseases that then need medications. Normal behavior is easily medicalized into an illness.

In fact, all of the hundreds of psychiatric diseases are arbitrary, man-made, and concocted. Any psychiatric diagnosis is made from the specialty's bible called the *Diagnostic and Statistical Manual of Mental Disorders* (*DSM–5*). Unlike other true diseases, which are verified by pathological findings, no doctor can look under a microscope or run a blood test to confirm that someone has a psychiatric disorder. The descriptions and definitions for psychiatric illnesses all come from panels of shrinks sitting in a room making up stuff.

Since the vague definitions of psychiatric illnesses can be applied to such a large portion of the population, that spells dollar signs for Big Pharma. Millions of perfectly normal people have been irreparably harmed by powerful antidepressants, antipsychotics, sedatives, and stimulants.

Depression and Bipolar

Despite "black box" warnings from the FDA on the drug labels that antidepressants increase the chance of suicide (and homicide as well, since many suicides are often associated with a simultaneous homicide event, but it would become a criminal matter for the FDA to sanction a murder-causing drug), or overall death (antipsychotics increase the risk of death in elderly, as well as cause diabetes), the shrinks still prescribe them like water. The psychiatry profession has utterly failed to regulate itself and weed out the bad doctors.

The main reason that suicide in the military is at an epidemic level, in my educated opinion, is because the military psychiatrists are the worst of the worst. They medicate any soldier who walks into their offices complaining of unhappiness or stress.[30] Likewise, the vast majority of young males who commit mass shootings at schools, etc. were also taking antidepressants. Those drugs clearly did not prevent the suicide/homicide event, and I argue that they pushed the patients over the edge to committing suicide.

Antidepressants selectively inhibit the reuptake of neurotransmitters, serotonin and norepinephrine, by the next neuron in line that would normally absorb them.[31] Keeping these neurotransmitters in play, the drugs constantly stimulate the brain, leading to euphoria. It is the same way that cocaine and amphetamines work.

But that false-high comes with a price. Eventually, the brain becomes exhausted of neurotransmitters and a tremendous gloom and depression onsets. That is why these horrible drugs do not help treat depression, but rather cause it.

---

[30] Cardin B, Greer SE. "Senator Ben Cardin discusses antidepressants in the military." *The Healthcare Channel* website. https://thehcc.tv December, 2009.

[31] Harner c, et al. "How do antidepressants work? New perspectives for refining future treatment approaches" *Lancet Psychiatry*. 2017 May; 4(5): 409–418.

Ponder this if you will: Vulnerable patients, often incorrectly diagnosed with depression by quacks, are given drugs that put them into a death spiral. Many of these patients are very young too. Only in the American healthcare system, where the industry lobbyists have corrupted the oversight agencies, such as the FDA, can bad drugs be used so commonly, with deadly consequences.

What I say is not controversial at all. There is a mountain of clinical trial evidence that backs me up. As I said, it is right there in the FDA warning labels.

The American Medical Association stated in 2012:

"In October of 2004, the Federal Drug Administration (FDA) issued a "black-box" label warning indicating that the use of certain antidepressants to treat major depressive disorder (MDD) in adolescents may increase the risk of suicidal ideations and behaviors. The warning came shortly after the FDA's British counterpart, the Medicines and Healthcare products Regulatory Agency (MHRA), concluded that selective serotonin reuptake inhibitors (SSRIs) with the exception of fluoxetine (Prozac) should not be used to treat adolescents with major depressive disorders.

The MHRA's 2003 recommendation, based on a report by the Committee on Safety of Medicines' Expert Working Group, states that, with the exception of fluoxetine, SSRIs have not been found efficacious in randomized clinical trials. Moreover, the group also noticed an increased risk of suicidal behaviors among adolescent patients being treated with

SSRIs and judged that the balance of risks and benefits did not favor the use of SSRIs for adolescents with MDD. Only fluoxetine showed significant therapeutic benefits; fluvoxamine (Luvox) lacked evidence to warrant any cost-benefit analysis."[32]

More recently the largest randomized-controlled trials of its kind, conducted in England, concluded that the most common antidepressant does not work at reducing depression.[33] "Its authors said they were "shocked and surprised" by the results, and called for the development of new classes of medication."[34]

ADHD

If you think I have strong opinions about antidepressants, then do not get me started on Attention-Deficit/Hyperactivity Disorder, or ADHD. At least depression is a genuine affliction in some cases. In contrast, ADHD is a relatively new man-made disease concocted by American psychiatrists and school teachers. Plenty of books by respected doctors say the same thing.[35]

---

[32] Ho D. "Antidepressants and the FDA's Black-Box Warning: Determining a Rational Public Policy in the Absence of Sufficient Evidence." *AMA Journ. Ethics. Virtual Mentor*. 2012;14(6):483-488.
[33] Lewis G, et al. "The clinical effectiveness of sertraline in primary care and the role of depression severity and duration (PANDA): a pragmatic, double-blind, placebo-controlled randomised trial" *Lancet Psychiatry*. Published online September 19, 2019. https://www.thelancet.com/journals/lanpsy/article/PIIS2215-0366(19)30366-9/fulltext
[34] Bodkin H. "Most common antidepressant barely helps improve depression symptoms, 'shocking' trial finds" *The Telegraph*. September 19, 2019.
[35] Saul R. "Doctor: ADHD Does Not Exist" *Time Magazine*. March, 2014.

For starters, ADHD is a uniquely American "disease" Only 0.5% of kids in France are diagnoses with ADHD and treated with drugs, for example. In the U.S., 9% kids are diagnoses with ADHD and treated with drugs.[36] That is a 17-fold, or 1,700%, increase in incidence, which is biologically implausible. Therefore, the definition and diagnosis are both flawed.

French doctors and teachers do not use the shrinks' bible, the DSM-5. They also look to solve the underlying problem causing the child to be hyperactive, then apply counseling, not drugs.

In the U.S., ADHD is an official disability recognized by the government. Therefore, schools receive funds for having ADHD students. Doped up and sedated kids are also easier to handle, pleasing the teachers' union. It does not even require a doctor to diagnose ADHD in the U.S. Teachers and counselors are usually the ones telling parents that their kid has ADHD.

ADHD drugs are highly addictive. They also alter the development of young brains. Patients taking ADHD stimulants develop depression and irritability, just like cocaine addicts.

Until 1959, benzadrine, also known as "bennies", was available without a prescription. Benzadrine is an amphetamine. Doctors finally realized that these stimulants were addictive and the drugs were taken off the market.

Well, decades later, the drug companies tweaked the molecules a bit and reintroduced amphetamines as ADHD treatments for children (i.e. Ritalin (methylphenidate), Adderall (amphetamine), etc.). The same drugs that helped kill Elvis, hooked Johnny Cash, and

---

[36] Wedge M. "Why French Kids Don't Have ADHD." *Psychology Today* website. https://www.psychologytoday.com March, 2018.

contributed to Hitler's insanity, are now being prescribed by quacks to toddlers for treatment of a bogus disease.

Gluten Intolerance

Over the last decade, mostly in coastal cities, millions of Americans think they now have a disease caused by a wheat protein called gluten. However, they are misguided. It is complete nonsense.[37]

Celiac disease is a rare disorder whereby intestinal tissue seems to be allergic to gluten. It was "discovered" in a very small trial of only a few dozen people. Even celiac disease is likely bogus. But for sure, the masses who now buy food because it is gluten-free are sheep following the lead of TV quacks like Dr. Oz. They do not have gluten-intolerance.

On my Healthcare Channel, I interviewed Alessio Fasano, MD, the Harvard doctor who started this fad accidentally.[38] Even he is appalled by what has become of the anti-gluten movement.

Restless Leg Syndrome

How far will Big Pharma go to medicalize normal behavior in order to make an excuse to sell a useless drug? The industry seems to have met the limits with restless leg syndrome.

---

[37] Croal I, et al. "Gluten Does Not Induce Gastrointestinal Symptoms in Healthy Volunteers: A Double-Blind Randomized Placebo Trial" *Gastroenterology*. September, 2019. Volume 157, Issue 3, Pages 881–883

[38] Fasano A, Greer SE. "The Hype Surrounding Gluten." *The Healthcare Channel* https://thehcc.tv 2014

Restless leg syndrome is laughably bogus. I can imagine it now. Some drug executive had a spouse who moved around a lot at night. He (likely a man) thought, "Wow. What if a I sedated her and then sold it as a new drug?"

In 2012, GlaxoSmithKline gave up on its partnership with small biotech company XenoPort for the development of a drug called Horizant to treat restless leg. The drug eventually made it to the market, but it is barely used. XenoPort was eventually sold for scrap value to another drug company.

People with restless legs exist by the millions, but what they suffer from is a sleep disorder. There are many reasons for people not achieve proper REM sound sleep.

Chapter 6. Unsafe Drugs and Medical Devices

In 1998, when I was still a surgery resident and conducting my multi-center randomized-controlled clinical trial[39] on a wound healing device known now as negative pressure therapy, I devised a better mousetrap, so to speak. I assembled a team that included an NYU Stern School of Business professor and we met with the heads Bristol-Myers Squibb's Convatec division.

Then, in 1999, I devised a breast reconstruction device and had prototypes built by Cook Medical in Indiana. I partnered with a prominent plastic surgeon who ran a hospital in Guadalajara, Mexico and flew there to implant the first-in-woman devices.

By that time, I knew I was interested in pursuing the business side of surgery. I left my NYU residency program, gave my federal research grant money to a friend in the plastic surgery program, and began working for the Wall Street bank *Donaldson, Lufkin, and Jenrette* (DLJ) as a medical device sell-side research analyst. The year was 2000. It was rare at the time for a medical doctor to go into Wall Street. There are now hundreds of MD's in the field.

DLJ was quickly acquired in my first year there by *Credit Suisse*. As an analyst at both banks, I wrote the reports and built the financial models for companies that

---

[39] Greer SE, et al. "Preliminary Results from a Multicenter, Randomized, Controlled, Study of the Use of Subatmospheric Pressure Dressing for Pressure Ulcer Healing." Accepted for presentation at the Joint Meeting of the European Tissue Repair Society and The Wound Healing Society. Bordeaux, France. August, 1999 (Of note, the trial was still underway at this time, but I had left for a career in Wall Street. I had handed off the well-funded prestigious trial to my colleagues at NYU, led by Michael Longaker, MD, but they were unable to complete it.)

we covered, such as Johnson & Johnson, Medtronic, Boston Scientific, Abbott, etc. Our team went along with the investment bankers to pitch private companies to use our bank to lead underwrite their IPOs, etc. (i.e. the "sell-side").

I left the sell-side after about a year and started to work for a hedge fund tycoon on the buy-side. I then became the portfolio manager for Merrill Lynch's internal hedge fund. I had $250 Million at my disposal to invest in publicly-traded stocks.

Investing might sound cushy and fun, but it is extremely stressful. One eats what they kill, so to speak. In order to make any money, equity investors must try to predict the future by studying the clinical trial data on drugs and devices, then handicap the odds of whether the FDA will approve them.

Analysts who have large sums of money on the line, betting one way or the other on the future of a drug or device, become far more versed in the data than a practicing doctor. This is how I gained so much insight.

I know where the bodies lie. I know which therapy is an ineffective scam and which ones should be used. I know the safety hazards that the industries downplay. I know how the drug and device companies give doctors kickbacks to use their products.

In short, nobody can spot corporate malfeasance in the healthcare sectors better than I can. I state that not to be arrogant, but rather to let you the reader understand my credentials.

Number Needed to Treat

A fancy biostatistical term that all patients should know about is the Number Needed to Treat (NNT). "The Number Needed to Treat (NNT) is the number of patients you need to treat to prevent one additional bad outcome (e.g. death, stroke, etc.). For example, if a drug has an NNT of 5, it means you have to treat 5 people with the drug to prevent one additional bad outcome."[40]

The bigger the number, the less effective is the therapy. If the NNT = 1, then every single patient is successfully treated. Many surgical procedures are highly effective with an NNT of nearly 1. However, most drugs are far less effective with large NNT.

Most Drugs and Medical Devices are Ineffective

Drugs and devices often have an NNT of more than 100, meaning they don't work worth a damn. Even when the desired outcome is reached, it is often clinically meaningless, such as a prolongation of the time a tumor stays small by three-months. Most cancer drugs do not actually prolong life, much less cure the patient. Cardiology drugs, such as statins, simply do not work at all in most patients, and so on.

However, far more likely of an outcome in America is an adverse event caused by a therapy. The probability of suffering an adverse event is many times that of the probability that the patient will benefit from the drug.

---

[40] "Number Needed to Treat (NNT)" *The Centre for Evidence-Based Medicine.* https://www.cebm.net/2014/03/number-needed-to-treat-nnt/

Despite these lopsided odds, ineffective and unsafe drugs and devices get approved by the FDA anyway. As previously discussed, the FDA has been thoroughly corrupted by industry dollars.

The Most Commonly Prescribed Drugs in America

Opioids Pain Pills

Vicodin (hydrocodone/acetaminophen) is the most commonly prescribed drug, despite it rarely having a proper indication for use. Most prescriptions are for long-term pain indications even though opioids are not meant for long-term pain management.[41] We now have an epidemic of opioid drug overdoses. More Americans die from overdoses each year (i.e. 70,000) than died in the entire 10-years of the Vietnam War.[42] Oh, by the way, the acetaminophen (generic name for Tylenol) in Vicodin is damaging to the liver when the addicts take large doses of the opioid.

Oxycontin (oxycodone), sold by Purdue Pharmaceuticals, is properly blamed for causing the opioid addition problem. I was in medical school in the 1990's when this started. Doctors were receiving lavish "educational dinners", then persuaded to treat all forms of pain with the strong addictive opioids. The drug marketing

---

[41] Dowell D, Greer SE. "The new CDC guidelines for prescribing opioid pain pills" *The Healthcare Channel*. June 1, 2016. https://thehcc.tv/2019/08/15/the-new-cdc-guidelines-for-prescribing-opioid-pain-pills/

[42] This was my novel observation and I relayed it to the Secretary of HHS and commissioner of the FDA. Then, President Trump made the same comment during his address to the nation from the Oval Office on January 8, 2019. Coincidence?

worked by creating a false epidemic of "untreated pain" Doctors were made to believe they were inhumane monsters of they did not prescribe pain pills to anyone who asked for them.

But what about the obvious addiction risks? Every doctor knows that opioids are addictive. Well, the drug industry created junk science that claimed the pain pills were not addictive. I was just a medical student at the time, and I knew it was a scam back then.

Purdue Pharmaceuticals company recently offered $12 Billion to settle hundreds of lawsuits. Yet no one has gone to jail despite perpetrating a mass murder. The Sackler family that owns Purdue are still among the richest people in the world.

The Washington Post investigated how all of these pain pills were getting into the hands of addicts. [43] They found that the big pharmacy names were knowingly shipping large volumes of opioid pills to small towns. From 2006 through 2012, 76-Billion pain pills were shipped.

The article states:

> "Just six companies distributed 75 percent of the pills during this period: McKesson Corp., Walgreens, Cardinal Health, AmerisourceBergen, CVS and Walmart, according to an analysis of the database by The Washington Post. Three companies manufactured 88 percent of the opioids: SpecGx, a subsidiary of

---

[43] Higham S, Horwitz S, et al. "76 billion opioid pills: Newly released federal data unmasks the epidemic" *Wash. Post.* July 16, 2019.

Mallinckrodt; Actavis Pharma; and Par Pharmaceutical, a subsidiary of Endo Pharmaceuticals. Purdue Pharma, which the plaintiffs allege sparked the epidemic in the 1990s with its introduction of OxyContin, its version of oxycodone, was ranked fourth among manufacturers with about 3 percent of the market.

The states that received the highest concentrations of pills per person per year were: West Virginia with 66.5, Kentucky with 63.3, South Carolina with 58, Tennessee with 57.7 and Nevada with 54.7. West Virginia also had the highest opioid death rate during this period. Rural areas were hit particularly hard: Norton, Va., with 306 pills per person; Martinsville, Va., with 242; Mingo County, W.Va., with 203; and Perry County, Ky., with 175."

The Washington Post article is based on federal DEA data. Our own protective agency knew all about this and did not act! The DEA fought The Post in court to prevent the data from being unsealed, but lost. Clearly, politicians receiving money from these companies, who influence what the DEA enforces, encouraged the agency to look the other way for decades.[44]

---

[44] Zezima K, et al. "As fentanyl deaths soared among their constituents, Congress failed to act despite dire warnings about the powerful opioid." *The Washington Post*. September 20, 2019.

The pain pill crisis exemplifies this double-edged sword of American medicine. Our doctors and companies are rewarded financially for innovating. But that same economic force leads to greed and corruption.

Cholesterol Lowering Drugs

Lipitor (atorvastatin) and Zocor (simvastatin) are two of the top-10 most commonly prescribed drugs. They are supposed to lower cholesterol and reduce clogged arteries.

However, statins simply do not work at all for most patients at low-risk for heart disease (i.e. primary prevention in patients who have never had a stroke, heart attack, or diabetes). Meanwhile, statins are indeed proven to cause muscle pain, liver damage, and increase the risk of developing diabetes.

Sanjay Kaul, MD of Cedars Sinai Hospital in Los Angeles, a frequent guest on my Healthcare Channel, has been a vocal critic of the overuse of statins in primary prevention. He has pointed out in numerous publications that the large industry-funded trials have been rigged to achieve the desired endpoints. The trials are usually stopped early, which is a well-known statistical scam to inflate efficacy and downplay adverse events. Also, the endpoints are meaningless composites of all sorts of outcomes predetermined to let the drug company put the thumb on the scale.

For example, in the 2011 AstraZeneca trial known as JUPITER, which studied Crestor (rosuvastatin), it was stopped prematurely under the excuse that the drug worked so well that it would have been unethical to continue to withhold it from the placebo group. Whenever you read that about a trial, be very skeptical. Also, what the study measured was a clinically meaningless "composite endpoint" Even with the trial rigged to win, the efficacy was low. However, when the low-risk patients were broken out, the drug did not show efficacy in that group.[45]

If one does a quick Internet search for the efficacy of statins, one is bombarded with meta-analyses and essays in journals showing that statins work even in the low-risk population. That is what billions and billions of dollars in drug revenue will produce. When all of the statistical tricks, such as early stoppage or composite endpoints, are dissected and forensically analyzed, the debilitating side effects and adverse events are not offset by the reduction in chance of death or heart attack.

In 2013, after the ACC and AHA changed the guidelines increasing the patient population eligible for statins to more than 40% of the adults in the country, backlash ensued. In 2018, those societies backed off somewhat on the idea that low-risk patients should be on statins based on some absurd, black-box, junk-science, "risk calculator" model[46], although the risk calculator still serves a vital function in the grand industrial propaganda scheme.[47] *"Vive la Risk-Calculator!"* the cardiology mafia from Boston chants.

[45] Kaul S. "Statins for Primary Prevention: Insights from JUPITER Trial", slides presented at CRT 2011 meeting, Washington DC. *CRTonline*.org http://www.crtonline.org/presentation-detail/statins-primary-prevention-insights-from-jupiter-t
[46] Krumholz H, Greer SE, "Can a "calculator" really tell doctors who should be on Lipitor?" *The Healthcare Channel*. November 13, 2013.
[47] Grundy S. "2018 AHA/ACC Guideline on the Management of Blood Cholesterol" *Circulation*. Vol. 139. No. 125. November, 2018.

Until Lipitor lost patent protection, it was the highest revenue drug in the world, earning $13-Billion a year at its peak. That allowed Pfizer to give most doctors in America some sort of kickback. AstraZeneca tried to take over where Lipitor left off with its Crestor drug scam, but it never materialized (in small part due to my reporting on The Healthcare Channel, Fox Business Network, and in the WSJ Health Blog).

Antibody Drugs That Lower Cholesterol

The good news is that there are indeed drugs very effective at lowering cholesterol. Repatha (evolocumab), made by Amgen, and Praluent (alirocumab), made by Sanofi and Regeneron, are the wonder drugs that the cardiology community wanted statins to be. They work so well that the atherosclerosis actually reverses and recedes.

So, why are few people taking these drugs? The companies tried to charge $10,000 per year for them. Given the millions of patients eligible, the insurance companies and Medicare restricted them.[48] The companies recently got smart and slashed the prices.

If you have high cholesterol and cannot tolerate statins, you should be on one of the drugs. But good luck. You will need a medical advocate to navigate the insurance companies.

---

[48] O'Neill W, Greer SE. "Insurance companies are not paying for Repatha and Praluent" *The Healthcare Channel*. March 12, 2017

Daily Aspirin

I was alarmed at the serious bleeding consequences of aspirin decades ago and become somewhat of an evangelical against the use of daily aspirin to supposedly prevent heart attacks. I then started to formally write short stories on my Healthcare Channel website that refuted the onslaught of junk science making it onto the mainstream TV news.

On CBS News, a shady doctor in California was starting to hype aspirin for cancer prevention too. I would counter each CBS News segment with a review of the literature and make sure that David Rhodes, the president of CBS News, read them.

Finally, a decade after I began my crusade, I was vindicated. In September of 2019, several large trials[49] were published in the New England Journal of medicine showing that daily aspirin did nothing to prevent heart attacks, but definitely did increase the risk of deadly bleeding into the brain and GI tract.

The major cardiology societies changed their guidelines, dropping daily aspirin. But the California doctor refused to throw in the towel on CBS.[50]

---

[49] McNeil J, et al. "Effect of Aspirin on Cardiovascular Events and Bleeding in the Healthy Elderly" *N Engl J Med* 2018; 379:1509-1518
[50] Greer SE. "TV Quack Dr. David Agus still likes daily aspirin despite heart guidelines dropping it." *The Healthcare Channel*. https://thehcc.tv 2019.

Blood Pressure Drugs

New guidelines from the Greek Gods of Medicine (i.e. the medical societies, such as the AHA and ACC) mean that 46% of American adults, or more than 100-Million Americans, should be on some form of high blood pressure medication. Prinivil or Zestril (lisinopril), Norvasc (amlodipine), and hydrochlorothiazide are three of the Top-10 most prescribed drugs. But—you guessed it—the drugs have little clinical trial data to show that they reduce blood pressure, and therefore, prevent kidney damage, stroke, etc.

The drug industry, which funds the medical societies that make the guidelines, keeps producing junk science that lowers the definition of "high blood pressure" The cutoff is now 130/80 mm Hg, down from 140/90.

To be sure, hypertension is deadly. It does wreak havoc on the delicate blood vessels in the kidneys, eyes, and brain. But American medicine is overtreating hypertension. Millions of Americans have numerous costly pills to take each day, which causes them to go to the bathroom too frequently or faint easily. It is debilitating to their quality of life.

Antibiotics

The Z-pack, or Zithromax, (azithromycin and amoxicillin) is among the Top-10 most prescribed drugs. By now, most people are aware that antibiotics are overprescribed. Yet doctors still do it.

Antibiotics are bad when consumed unnecessarily because they can cause disruptions in the normal flora of bacterium we all have, particularly in the colon. When normal bacterium are killed off by antibiotics, dangerous other bacterium then multiply. Clostridium difficile, or "C.

diff", can damage the lining of the colon causing diarrhea, dehydration, and death. However, despite C. diff being a big problem for hospitals, doctors still place many patients on powerful IV antibiotics when it is not necessary.

Antidepressants and Antipsychotics

In a JAMA report, 12% of the 244 adults in America, or 30 million, were taking antidepressants, and 17% were on some form of psychiatric drug. [51] Those were defined as being either antidepressants, anxiolytics (sedatives and hypnotics), or antipsychotics.

The numbers become more startling when the young child population is studied. According to data from a company that tracks real prescriptions, 7.2 million kids aged from 0 to 5 were on one of the psychiatric drugs listed above, or a stimulant much like methamphetamine or cocaine to treat Attention Deficit and Hyperactivity Disorder (ADHD). [52]

Brains in children this small are still developing and these powerful drugs permanently alter the brains. [53] But there certainly is a good reason then for respected MDs to

---

[51] Moore T, et al. "Adult Utilization of Psychiatric Drugs and Differences by Sex, Age, and Race" *JAMA Intern Med.* 2017;177(2):274-275

[52] "Number of Children & Adolescents Taking Psychiatric Drugs in the U.S." *The Citizens Commission on Human Rights.* https://www.cchrint.org/psychiatric-drugs/children-on-psychiatric-drugs/

[53] Bouziane C, et al. "White Matter by Diffusion MRI Following Methylphenidate Treatment: A Randomized Control Trial in Males with Attention-Deficit/Hyperactivity Disorder" Radiology. Published online August 13, 2019. Not yet in print. https://pubs.rsna.org/doi/10.1148/radiol.2019182528

prescribe powerful drugs to these little angels. The clinical evidence must be overwhelming, right?

Well—shocker—there are no such data. In fact, the entire "disease" of ADHD is a concocted manmade joke recognized only by American doctors. European kids do not have an epidemic of ADHD, as I previously discussed.

Caffeine

Caffeine is a potent drug, but few think of it that way. It is in or sodas, coffee, and tea. Diet pills are caffeine.

It seems that every week the mainstream TV news runs with some junk-science report funded by the coffee industry claiming that coffee is good for you. But those claims are totally bogus.

For people who drink many cups of coffee a day, they develop heart dysrhythmias, such as premature ventricular contraction (PVCs). They develop psychiatric illnesses ranging from moodiness to paranoia. It also stains the teeth and causes kidney stones.

Just do an Internet search of "Is coffee good for you?" and you will find one "large study" after the other that concludes coffee does everything from prolong lifespan to reduce cancer. There are "studies" that deny the adverse events caused by caffeine. But every single one of these studies are simply meta-analyses, where a bunch of small junk-studies are combined to get an even bigger junk-study. Moreover, the groups publishing the studies are funded by coffee industry grants. The bottom line is that there has never been a properly conducted, reputable, randomized-controlled-study showing that coffee is good for you.[54]

For years, I would complain to the president of CBS News, David Rhodes, that the latest coffee "research" they constantly touted was erroneous industry-funded propaganda. I have no doubt that these TV "news" shows receive funding from publicists in exchange for running these fake stories.

I was finally vindicated in 2018 when California mandated cancer warnings be placed on coffee due to the carcinogenic nature of the acrylamide in it. The response by the CBS morning crew was priceless.[55]

Whether or not coffee causes cancer is not the critical question. Without a doubt, we know that caffeine raises blood pressure, alters the normal heart rhythms (i.e. causes dysrhythmias), and creates irritability when taken at large doses daily, as many Americans do.

I personally drink a cup of coffee a day, but as a pure luxury. I like the smell and flavor of it. I roast my own beans at home and use the pour-over technique for brewing. It is a delicacy for me.

But when I was in Wall Street, stressed out to the max, drinking coffee all day long, I started to develop bad PVC's. One weekend, I was taking a nap because I was chronically exhausted. I was awakened in my Manhattan high-rise by what I thought was an earthquake rocking the building. It was my heart pounding from PVC's.

---

[54] For more information, go to The Healthcare Channel at https://thehcc.tv/ and search "coffee"
[55] Greer SE. "CBS News not happy at all that cancer warning added to coffee." *The Healthcare Channel.* 2018 https://thehcc.tv/

That is one reason I left the investment industry (the other being that my type of job was replaced by computer algorithms, exchange-traded funds, and high-speed trading strategies). Stress is a killer. People who are constantly sleep-deprived and stressed have high levels of cortisol and other harmful hormones. Those elevate the blood pressure and increase hunger. Stressed out people eat a lot because of these hormones.

Coffee is the gateway drug to this cascade of stressful evets. The caffeine causes stress. We then eat more, particularly sugary foods, because of the stress. A Starbucks latte is nothing but a milkshake with caffeine. The obesity that ensues then makes us exhausted and sleep-deprived. And finally, people then turn to cigarettes or cocaine to wake up and get through the day.

Nothing exemplifies this better than a Wall Street biotech analyst I once knew. He was an MD from Johns Hopkins and very good at his job. He was a nerdy little guy. When he spoke to investors on conference calls or videos, he was always hyped up from coffee, I thought. He then lost his job due to rumored cocaine and/or opioid addiction. He died in August of 2019 at the age of 46. One can only speculate as to the cause of death.

I am not blaming caffeine for this man's ultimate demise. I am simply pointing out that caffeine is an unhealthy crutch to maintain untenable lifestyles. Find out why you need coffee in the afternoon, or why are you not sleeping well.

The Most Profitable Drugs in America

The drugs listed above are the most commonly prescribed or used, but they are not the most profitable.

That award goes to a group of outrageously expensive drugs that are—you guessed it again—often ineffective and also dangerous.

Humira and Enbrel

Humira (adalimumab) and Enbrel (etanercept) are what is called "biologics" They are bioengineered antibodies designed to attack a molecule called Tumor Necrosis Factor (TNF). Part of the normal inflammation cycle, when run amok, TNF is what damages a patient's own cells, to cause rheumatoid arthritis, psoriasis, and other diseases.

These anti-TNF drugs are effective at stopping arthritis and psoriasis, but they are also deadly. By stopping the normal immune system, cancers grow. Lymphoma is stated in the FDA-approved "black box" warning labels of these drugs.

That is right: Drugs that cause cancer are also the most profitable drugs in America.

Because of this profit, and the money that trickles down to doctors, the risks of these drugs are not discussed properly with patients. The true risk-benefit analysis is not made known in most cases.

Is unsightly skin psoriasis worth risking developing lymphoma or infectious diseases? You could ask Glenn Frey of The Eagles if he were alive. He was on Humira and died from opportunist infections.[56]

---

[56] Fears D. "The dark side of the arthritis drug blamed in Glenn Frey's death" *New York Post*. January 20, 2016.

Eliquis and Xarelto

Eliquis (apixaban), made by Bristol-Meyers Squibb, and Xarelto (rivaroxoban), made by Johnson & Johnson, are new forms of blood thinners given to patients who have coronary conditions that place them at high-risk for stroke due to blood clots inside the heart. They were approved by the FDA to supposedly be safer ways to thin the blood than inexpensive warfarin.

In less than a decade, these costly drugs have become widely prescribed. Eliquis earns about $8-Billion a year for Bristol-Meyers Squibb, and that is growing at 30%. Xarelto earns about $2-Billion for Johnson & Johnson and is losing out to Eliquis. Pradaxa (dabigatran) by Boehringer Ingelheim Pharmaceuticals earns about $2-Billion as well.

Is the cost worth it? Are fewer people suffering strokes?

By now, you know that all of these questions are rhetorical. Of course, there are few data showing that these new drugs have helped to reduce stroke any better than the generic warfarin.

In 2011, the big Bristol-Meyers Squibb trial that goes by the acronym ARISTOTLE supposedly showed that Eliquis reduced more stroke than generic warfarin (i.e. also known as the original brand name of Coumadin, warfarin is the same drug used as rat poison). But large industry-funded studies like these are usually highly misleading.

While on Wall Street, I became an expert at forensically debunking them. They are rigged to succeed and meet the endpoints, as I mentioned. The definitions of the outcomes, or the endpoints, are commonly clinically meaningless. The adverse events, such as stroke, are often defined subjectively. What exactly is a "stroke"? The patients studied are mostly enrolled from other parts of the world where tight oversight is impossible, such as Eastern Europe, India, or Africa. Those patients are not North American and have different genetic profiles and lifestyles, thus making them often unreliable as test subjects for drugs that will be used in North America. And the statistics are almost always manipulated.

In 2018, a study published in *Stroke*[57] looked at the real-world use of Eliquis. The drug did not reduce stroke any better than warfarin. It did have fewer cases of deadly bleeding, however. But, because of the ARISTOTLE trial and subsequent FDA label that claims it is a better drug than the others, Eliquis has cleaned house, dominating the market.

I can only imagine how many doctors have had their travel to medical meetings paid for by Bristol-Meyers Squibb and Pfizer. Eight-Billion-dollars pays for a lot of "medical education"

Cancer Drugs

Cancer: nobody wants to get cancer. But the detrimental effects of the diseases collectively known as cancer are just part of the suffering that a cancer patient will suffer. For reasons discussed more later, the drugs prescribed by oncologists are determined in part by the amount of profit they generate for the doctor. Oncology is

---

[57] Proietti M, et al. "Real-World Use of Apixaban for Stroke Prevention in Atrial Fibrillation: A Systematic Review and Meta-Analysis" *Stroke*. 2018 Jan;49(1):98-106.

the only medical specialty where it is legal for the doctor's office or hospital to charge a markup on the base cost of the drugs. Therefore, the costlier the drug, the more the doctor makes.

With these perverse market forces, and a total fear by any politician of being smeared by the drug industry as an impediment to cancer victims receiving life-saving care, and laws that forbid Medicare from fighting price gouging, greedy drug companies are charging more than $100,000 a year for the new cancer drugs. Some are now priced at $1 million per patient. President Trump has been vocal about high drug prices, and the companies openly defy him.

Drugs that are Under-Prescribed

So far, I have talked about drugs and devices that are overutilized in America, primarily for financial profit reasons. Well, the converse is occasionally true as well. There are some inexpensive drugs (thus unprofitable for the drug companies) that are not prescribed as much as they should be.

Just as any of the ineffective drugs I previously mentioned are prescribe far too often because the drug companies give financial incentives to doctors and spend billions on marketing to the consumer, so too are effective generic drugs off the radar of doctors and ignored because there is no such marketing campaign associated with them.

Sadly, one would think that medical school and residency training would train doctors to know which medications work and which ones do not. But that does not happen.

Peer pressure is a real force seen in academic medicine. What do you think all of those high-brow medical society meetings, funded by the drug company, are for? They set the stage for what all good doctors should be doing, or so they are brainwashed.

However, most doctors do not have a clue about the efficacy or the real side effects of the drugs they use. They prescribe them because everyone else is doing it. Very few doctors read the medical literature, and fewer still know how to spot junk science.

Estrogen Replacement Therapy

The majority of post-menopausal women should be taking some form of hormone replacement therapy (HRT), whether it be estrogen with progesterone or estrogen alone. The drugs are generic and cheap. I have been telling this to anyone who listens for decades.

Yet almost no American doctor prescribes them. Why? HRT is rarely prescribed because some poorly conducted studies (and even more poorly interpreted by the medical societies) in the late 1990's and early 2000's concluded that HRT raised the risk of heart attack and breast cancer.[58,59,60,61]

---

[58] Hulley S, et al. "Randomized trial of estrogen plus progestin for secondary prevention of coronary heart disease in postmenopausal women" *JAMA* 1998; 280: 605-13.

[59] Rossouw JE, et al. "Risks and benefits of estrogen plus progestin in healthy postmenopausal women: principal results from the Women's Health Initiative randomized controlled trial" *JAMA* 2002; 288: 321-33.

[60] Manson JE, Hsia J, Johnson KC, et al. "Estrogen plus progestin and the risk of coronary heart disease" *N Engl J Med* 2003; 349: 523-34.

[61] Anderson GL, et al. "Effects of conjugated equine estrogen in postmenopausal women with hysterectomy: the Women's Health Initiative randomized controlled trial" *JAMA* 2004; 291: 1701-12.

However, I had spent an entire year during medical school researching estrogen on a hairless mouse model.[62] Clinically, I saw the dramatic effects on women of the loss of estrogen. Their skin becomes thinner (i.e. the subject of my research in medical school)(If you look at any Hollywood actress over 60-years-old who still looks great, the chances are that they are on HRT), bones become brittle, and muscle wastes away. Those are the important symptoms to monitor. But instead, HRT is thought of only as a therapy to prevent hot flashes.

When the landmark studies against the use of HRT caused doctors to be afraid to prescribe it, I was a Wall Street analyst by then. I looked at the studies and quickly saw the design flaws. I have been advocating for HRT for almost two-decades as the entire medical world was doing the opposite.

Was I a quack all this time? Nope. I was finally vindicated in 2016 by a New England Journal of Medicine paper,[63] which reversed the dogma that HRT was deadly.

The authors concluded:

> "Oral estradiol therapy was associated with less progression of subclinical atherosclerosis than was placebo when therapy was initiated within 6 years after menopause but not when it was initiated 10 or more years after menopause.

---

[62] Greer SE, et al. "The Effects Of Estrogen on Photoaged Skin and Chemical Peeling" Presented at the 1994 William H. Saunders Lectureship, The Ohio State University College of Medicine. Columbus, Ohio.

[63] Hodis HN, et al. "Vascular effects of early versus late postmenopausal treatment with Estradiol" *N Engl J Med.* 2016;374(13):1221-1231.

Estradiol had no significant effect on cardiac CT measures of atherosclerosis in either postmenopause stratum."

In other words, in this newer randomized-controlled trial, HRT was not only safe, but it reduced the chance of hardening of the arteries.

Then, a year later in 2017, Harvard researcher JoAnn Manson, MD, who was one of the authors of the original papers warning about HRT, did a 180-degree turn and concluded in a paper in JAMA[64] that, after further study, they were dead wrong. Oops.

Those authors concluded:

"Among postmenopausal women, hormone therapy with CEE plus MPA for a median of 5.6 years or with CEE alone for a median of 7.2 years was not associated with risk of all-cause, cardiovascular, or cancer mortality during a cumulative follow-up of 18 years."

I went into some wonky detail over estrogen and HRT to show you how this all works. Doctors have a simple task to do, which is to critically read (i.e. not to assume it is gospel) the medical literature, but almost none of them do so. As a result, in this case of HRT, hundreds of millions of American women alone, not to mention the rest of the world, were deprived of life-saving drugs that also improve quality of life.

---

[64] Manson JE, et al. "Menopausal hormone therapy and long-term all-cause and cause-specific mortality: The Women's Health Initiative randomized trials" *JAMA*. doi:10.1001/jama.2017.11217

By the way, my own mother is a victim of this. She understandably chose to listen to her primary care doctor who decided to not prescribe HRT. After the first paper in 2016, I informed him of it and he made no change in his clinical practice, because his peers were not changing.

To this day, despite many other large studies vindicating HRT, most doctors will not prescribe it due to peer pressure and dogma. However, you can bet your britches that HRT would be one of the most heavily marketed and prescribed drugs if it were patent-protected and able to make billions of dollars.

Drug Price Gouging

Since the new antibody drugs, such as Humira, Enbrel, and Avastin, were approved by the FDA in the early 2000's, the drug companies have been unable, for the most part, to invent new drugs that help large portions of the population (i.e. blockbuster drugs). The glory days of Lipitor were never recreated.

Despite that, drug company profits keep rising. That is because they simply hike the prices. In no other sector of the economy does one see this price inelasticity, or ability to hike the price of a product year after year, at a rate of 10% or more, and not lose demand. How does Big Pharma get away with it?

Part of the problem is that healthcare services and products are not directly purchased by the end-user. This third-party-payer problem creates price inflation.

Drug price inflation is greater than the rest of healthcare inflation. Overall, National Healthcare Expenditure is growing at about 5%. However, drug prices are growing at an inflation rate of 9% to 15%.[65] The price of drugs to treat rare diseases is growing at 20% per year.

Even generic drugs, once thought of as costing just a few bucks, are growing at 5%, or much higher than the overall inflation of the American economy. But some have gone up astronomical amounts once the producers cornered the market.

I was the very first person in the media to expose this generic drug scam of cornering the market and then hiking prices. Way back in 2009, my mother saw that her ear drops, once costing a few bucks, now cost her hundreds. I wrote a story on my Healthcare Channel to explain that the price hike was 1000%.[66] Everyone outside of a select group of the best Wall Street analysts ignored me.

Then, in 2015, "Pharma Bro" Martin Shkreli made the news for cornering the market on a life-saving HIV drug called Daraprim. His Turing Pharmaceuticals hiked the price 5,700%. He was later convicted of financial fraud and sits in federal prison now. But Shkreli only went to prison because he foolishly mocked congress. Had he just stayed quiet, he would have gotten away with this crime like all of the other companies have.

Drug companies are hiking prices to absurd levels because they can. Arcane laws written by lobbyists prohibit Medicare from negotiating prices. Congress is in the pocket of Big Pharma, so the laws will not be rescinded. Even

[65] Hernandez I, et al. "The Contribution Of New Product Entry Versus Existing Product Inflation In The Rising Costs Of Drugs." *Health Affairs.* Vol. 38, No. 1: January, 2019.
[66] Greer SE. "Actavis 1000% drug price hike: a case for healthcare reform." *The Healthcare Channel.* May 26, 2009.

President Trump, a man who takes pride in following through on his threats, and who has made high drug prices a priority, cannot stop the price gouging.

Unsafe Medical Devices

Medical devices are a topic that I know more about than most any other doctor. As a surgeon, I use them and see others using them. Then, as a Wall Street analyst, I covered the companies that make them. In the course of doing that, I had to learn the clinical data that supported the FDA approval process, among other things.

The FDA approval process for drugs has been watered down by the lobbyists, but the approval process for most medical devices is far worse. It requires nothing but filling out forms and paying fees in a "510(k)" process. For the rare instances where human clinical trials are required by the FDA, such as devices that go into the heart, the trials are poorly designed with short follow-up and clinically meaningless endpoints.

Currently, the only way to know whether the devices are safe is by monitoring real patients who act as guinea pigs. Even then, reporting of events where medical devices malfunction or were otherwise unsafe is not mandatory, and the reports are often ignored by the FDA.

For example, back in the 2000's, the large doses of radiation delivered by CT-scans was a concern to FDA scientists. But the medical device section leader of the FDA retaliated against the scientists.[67] Their computers were spied on and the scientists were eventually fired.

---

[67] "FDA suppressed CT safety concerns: scientist" *The Associated Press.* March 31, 2010. https://www.cbc.ca/news/technology/fda-suppressed-ct-safety-concerns-scientist-1.868102

This type of response by the divisional heads of the FDA, who are in the pockets of the medical device industry, is far too common. Although it is a smaller industry than Big Pharma, the medical device lobbyists have been notoriously powerful in Washington.

Hip and knee implants should be so important to get right that clinical trials would be required before approval, one would think. But no. They get approved by the 510(k) process. So, not surprisingly, many instances of unsafe implants have occurred. Metal-on-metal hips released cobalt micro-particles that caused constant inflammation and then cancers.[68] I spotted this safety concern back in the early 2000's when I was writing the reports on the orthopedic industry for Wall Street research firm *Sanford Bernstein*. A decade later, it all became widely known.

Implantable cardioverter defibrillators (ICDs) are devices also approved by the 510(k). This is despite these devices going inside the heart, with lots of parts that can fail, and many models having a track record of causing serious harm. For example, the wires that screw into the inside wall of the heart can poke through the heart or fracture.

I was the healthcare portfolio manager at Merrill Lynch in 2005 when Johnson & Johnson made a $25 billion offer to buy ICD-maker Guidant. Rarely do deals like this not happen once announced. But I knew that the Guidant devices were unsafe. Sure enough (and perhaps because of my activist investing) the deal was cancelled,

---

[68] "Metal-on-Metal Hip Implants" *The Food and Drug Administration* website. No Date. https://www.fda.gov/medical-devices/implants-and-prosthetics/metal-metal-hip-implants

sending Guidant shares down (I was short the stock and made millions for my portfolio.).

More recently, as coronary stents have become used less due to the very same safety issues that I first warned about in 2003, the interventional cardiologists are trying to fill the void with a new technology called Transcatheter Aortic Valve Replacement (TAVR). During the 2011 FDA panel meeting to determine whether TAVR devices should be approved, I spoke to the advisory panel pointing out the serious deficiencies in the trials.[69]

Traditional heart valves that are implanted by heart surgeons during open-heart surgery have many years of safety follow-up. That is because heart valves open and close millions of times and a failure is deadly to the patient. Man-made heart valves need long-term testing.

Well, the interventional cardiology mafia, as I call them, who are not heart surgeons, used their lobbying clout to get the FDA to approve TAVR valves with only one-year of clinical trial follow-up. The leader of that advisory panel was Harvard cardiologist William Maisel. Then, likely as a reward for allowing TAVR to pass through with a positive vote, he got a cushy job at the FDA. The industry likes him so much that he was able to survive a conviction of soliciting a prostitute and keep his job.[70]

Of course, all of the valve malfunction problems that I warned about are being seen in real-world applications. Astronaut and U.S. Senator John Glenn suffered a stroke after TAVR and died shortly thereafter.

---

[69] Greer SE. "The Only Five-Minutes of the Edwards Sapien AdCom You Need to Watch" *The Healthcare Channel.* July 28, 2011.
[70] Greer SE. "FDA official, William Maisel, pleads guilty to crime, keeps job" *The Healthcare Channel.* https://thehcc.tv

Thousands of others have to rely on pacemakers as a result of a TAVR adverse event, to name just a few.

William Boden, MD, a cardiologist and critic of many medical devices, stated, "It's a (redacted) joke. Once the COURAGE and BARI-2D trials showed that PCI (i.e. stenting) didn't reduce death or MI, the interventional cardiology community decided to re-invent themselves by creating a new subspecialty in "structural heart disease" (e.g. TAVRs, Mitral valve clips, PFO closure devices, left atrial appendage occlusion devices, etc.). With most of this stuff, they gloss over the complications ("it's the price of innovation") and the fact that outcomes are not durable. Some of these TAVR devices migrate a bit below the aortic valve plane and may block the ostia/openings of the coronary arteries, leading to ischemia or MI. As one aggressive interventionalist once opined, "There's not a cardiac condition for which a device doesn't exist""

As a final example, you probably think that contact lenses on the eye would be rigorously tested before the FDA approves them. Of course, that is not the case either. They are just 510(k).

I personally suffered a bad eye irritation many years back and tried to report it to the maker, Johnson & Johnson. They blew me off. At about this time was a national safety problem of serious infections caused by bad contact lens water solutions. I investigated and found that the FDA ignores consumer complaints.[71]

---

[71] Greer SE. "The inadequate FDA medical device safety surveillance system: a case study" *The Healthcare Channel.* https://thehcc.tv January 25, 2012.

Why are such dangers overlooked by hospitals and the FDA? It is all about money in Washington. The fees that hospitals earn from implanting these devices comprise a large portion of their overall revenue. The fees that the orthopedic surgeons, neurosurgeons, heart surgeons, cardiologists, and radiologists collect for themselves make them millionaires. If a hospital were to hassle them for implanting too many devices in patients that did not need the procedures, the doctors would walk across the street and work for another hospital.

Greed has corrupted many aspects of the caregiving process. As a medical advocate, I help patients avoid these pitfalls from unsafe and/or unnecessary medical devices.

Conflicts of Interest Between Your Doctor and Industry

In 2008, I started to help Senator Chuck Grassley with his efforts to protect whistleblowers. I had exposed some scandals related to the American College of Cardiology and the New York cardiology mafia.[72,73] That led to my slight assistance with Senator Grassley's efforts to create the Physician Payments Sunshine Act (PPS), which finally became law in 2010 as part of Obamacare.

---

[72] "Grassley, Kohl seek information about money going from medical device makers to doctors" The United States Senate Committee o Finance. October 16, 2018.
https://www.finance.senate.gov/ranking-members-news/grassley-kohl-seek-information-about-money-going-from-medical-device-makers-to-doctors
[73] Goldstein J. "Senators Probe Cardiologists' Ties to Stent Makers" *WSJ Health Blog*. October 16, 2008.
https://blogs.wsj.com/health/2008/10/16/senators-probe-cardiologists-ties-to-stent-makers/

The PPS makes public the payments from drug and device industries to medical doctors.

The PPS was fought staunchly and did not become active until 2013. Why did the industry fear this? The drug and device industries cannot get their products prescribed or implanted unless the MD gatekeepers sign off. How do they do that? They bribe them, of course.

The companies have created clever ways to funnel money to doctors without calling them kickbacks, which are illegal. It started with simple "educational" dinners, or paid "speaking engagements", that were nothing but vacations to ski resorts, etc. Then, it became so perverted that the companies selling big ticket items, such as orthopedic implants, would purchase vacation homes for surgeons. This is what led to the PPS.

The doctors prescribing the ultra-expensive drugs get similar kickbacks. However, oncologists are legally allowed to take a percentage of revenue from the overall price of the cancer drugs. Therefore, the more expensive the drug, the more likely it will be prescribed.

Fortunately, most doctors are just underpaid, overworked, schmucks not receiving significant payments from industry. But the more famous a doctor is as a "thought leader" at some big medical center, the more likely they are to be on the take.

Chapter 7. American Healthcare Harms You

Accidentally or intentionally, you can be harmed in many ways by the American medical system. Medical errors and unnecessary tests or procedures are also a common harm.

Medical Errors

Medical errors leading to serious adverse events are a problem much larger than most patients and doctors realize. Preventing them is a main goal of our medical advocacy service.

Twenty-years ago, the Institute of Medicine (IOM) released a seminal report called *To Err is Human*.[74] It studied the problem of medical mistakes and concluded that 100,000 patients a year are killed by them each year. That was more than the deaths caused by motor vehicle accidents, cancer, or AIDS at the time. But those statistics were low-balling the problem, assuming only 16% of hospital patients are victims to error. In reality, we now think that the rate is closer to 40%.[75]

That IOM report stated:

> "Yet silence surrounds this issue. For the most part, consumers believe they are protected. Media coverage has been limited to reporting of anecdotal cases. Licensure

---

[74] Kohn LT, et al. "To Err is Human: Building a Safer Health System" Institute of Medicine (US) Committee on Quality of Health Care in America. Washington (DC): *National Academies Press*; 2000.
[75] Makary M, et al. "Medical error—the third leading cause of death in the US" *BMJ*. 2016 ;353:i2139

and accreditation confer, in the eyes of the public, a "Good Housekeeping Seal of Approval." Yet, licensing and accreditation processes have focused only limited attention on the issue, and even these minimal efforts have confronted some resistance from health care organizations and providers. Providers also perceive the medical liability system as a serious impediment to systematic efforts to uncover and learn from errors.

The decentralized and fragmented nature of the health care delivery system (some would say "nonsystem") also contributes to unsafe conditions for patients, and serves as an impediment to efforts to improve safety. Even within hospitals and large medical groups, there are rigidly-defined areas of specialization and influence. For example, when patients see multiple providers in different settings, none of whom have access to complete information, it is easier for something to go wrong than when care is better coordinated. At the same time, the provision of care to patients by a collection of loosely affiliated organizations and providers makes it difficult to implement improved clinical information systems capable of providing timely access to complete patient information. Unsafe care is one of the prices we pay for not having organized systems of care with clear lines of accountability."

What exactly is a "medical error" as studied? The report stated, "According to noted expert James Reason, errors depend on two kinds of failures: either the correct action does not proceed as intended (an error of execution) or the original intended action is not correct (an error of planning). Errors can happen in all stages in the process of care, from diagnosis, to treatment, to preventive care."

Errors of execution are more challenging to prevent. Mistakes at the hands of the doctor during a procedure are not preventable, for the most part, other than to assure that the doctors undergo proper training. To err is human, as the IOM mentioned.

Hospitals can place signs all over stating that hand washing is mandatory, but they become quickly ignored, etc. Surgery departments can have weekly morbidity and mortality conferences, but true reasons for the mistakes are covered up and adverse events are not reduced. Hospitals and doctors get paid regardless of the quality of outcome.

Former John Hopkins researcher, Peter Pronovost MD PhD, proposed a radical idea in 2001 to implement pre-procedure checklists, just like the aviation industry uses.[76] Human memory is the biggest cause of errors. What we think is obvious can be overlooked or forgotten. The real-world application of his ideas dramatically reduced the rate of infection caused by central venous catheters.

---

[76] Pronovost P, et al. "An intervention to decrease catheter-related bloodstream infections in the ICU". *N. Engl. J. Med.* 355 (26): 2725–32. December, 2006

Then, Harvard researcher and surgeon, Atul Gawande MD, used checklists in the operating room.[77] If you have had any medical procedure lately, you likely noticed that the entire room of healthcare providers became very serious and started to verbally run down a checklist right before you went to sleep. The goal is to prevent horrible mistakes, such as removing the wrong limb, or even operating on the wrong patient entirely.

But errors of execution are still a huge problem. The Mount Carmel hospital chain in Central Ohio is a textbook example. They allegedly had a psychopath serial killer doctor named William Husel who allegedly murdered dozens of people by prescribing huge doses of fentanyl and other opioids. He was arrested, allowed to go free on bail, and awaits trial on 25-counts of murder. That was "error of intent" to be sure.

But the bigger story is how the madman doctor was able to affect his goal of overdoses. From the time a prescription is entered into the hospital electronic medical record system, then filled in the pharmacy, then delivered to the nursing station to be administered to the patient, there are supposed to be numerous safety check points. As a resident, I would occasionally make a mistake on the dose of an antibiotic, for example, and I would get a call from the pharmacist.

Yet, despite these built-in safety stops, Mount Carmel's system still allowed dozens of overdoses to happen. The CEO and many other employees ultimately got fired. This should have been the big story covered by journalist, but it was not.

---

[77] Gawande A. "The Checklist Manifesto: How to Get Things Right" Picador. 2011.

In contrast, unlike those errors of execution cited above, errors of planning (i.e. the competency of the doctor and staff) are more preventable if the patient has a medical advocate. Incorrect diagnoses, unnecessary drugs or surgeries, and suboptimal bedside nursing care can be avoided.

Second-Opinions

Although the American medical system acknowledges that second-opinions from other doctors are beneficial to outcome, in reality, few patients have the ability to get a proper, unbiased, second-opinion. A study[78] found that 20% of patients seek a second opinion, and this increases to 50% for cancer patients.[79]

Not only can a diagnosis be incorrect, but the plan of treatment often includes unnecessary tests and procedures. A Mayo Clinic study found that 88% of second opinions resulted in a different diagnosis. [80] Another study concluded, "Patient-initiated second opinions led to recommended changes in diagnosis for about 15%, and changes in treatment for about 37% of participants."[81]

---

[78] Wagner TH, et al. "Who gets second opinions?" *Health Aff* (Millwood). 1999 Sep-Oct;18(5):137-45.

[79] Hewitt M, et al. "Cancer prevalence and survivorship issues: analyses of the 1992 National Health Interview Survey." *J Natl Cancer Inst.* 1999 Sep 1;91(17):1480-6.

[80] Van Such, M, et al. "Extent of diagnostic agreement among medical referrals" *J Eval Clin Pract.* 2017; 23: 870– 874.

[81] Meyer a, et al. "Evaluation of Outcomes From a National Patient-initiated Second-opinion Program." *Am. Journ. Med*, Vol 128, No 10, October 2015

Help navigating this maze to get to the correct diagnosis and treatment is what our medical advocacy offers. Most medical centers have gotten in on the second-opinion racket because insurance and Medicare reimburses for second-opinions. But those doctors providing the second-opinion have conflicts of interest. There is a financial incentive to dismiss the first diagnosis and try to persuade the patient to come to their center of care instead. Getting a second diagnosis without an unbiased medical advocate can lead to more confusion rather than clarity.

A few years ago, my mother had a limp. She also had some back pain. I foolishly allowed her to see a spine surgeon at a major medical center. Sure enough, she left with a diagnosis of a bad back and spine surgery was planned.

Fortunately, my mother was her own advocate. Her instincts told her not to trust that surgeon and she saw another orthopedic team at a different medical center. It turned out that she had obvious osteoarthritis of the knee. A successful knee replacement cured her pain. Had she gotten the unnecessary spinal fusion surgery, she would have then needed a knee operation later.

The doctor who referred my mother and I to this spine surgeon was none other than the medical director. We went to medical school together. He was a trusted source and in charge of the place, yet still led us astray. He was not being malicious. He was simply doing what all good medical center employees do, which is to refer to their own doctors and assume that good care will be provided.

After that learning experience, my father also developed knee pain. He had no history of knee pain or arthritis before. He went straight to the same knee surgeon who cured my mother. Of course, he left with a diagnosis of osteoarthritis and knee surgery was planned.

Doctors do what they know best. They treat patients using their tools in their medical and cannot see outside of their professional training bubble. To a spine surgeon, all pain is spinal. To the hip and knee surgeon, all pain is from osteoarthritis, etc.

However, this time around, I was wiser and acted as his second-opinion doctor. We questioned the useless knee injections of hyaluronic acid that he was receiving. I was skeptical that he suddenly developed true knee arthritis. You don't just wake up one day with knee arthritis.

Then, after weeks of knee-injections and a knee surgery scheduled soon, my father's knee pain went away. It turns out that he had just sprained his knee ligaments shoveling snow. No knee surgery was required.

It makes the hair on the back of my neck stand up to think how close both of my parents came to becoming victims of the American medical system. It is not enough to get a second-opinion. One needs a medical advocate aligned with the patient's best interest, not aligned with the profit of the hospital or their personal practice.

Overused Diagnostic Tests and Imaging

As I laid out above, our fee-for-service healthcare system motives doctors and hospitals to perform unnecessary tests and procedures. I will list some of the most common ones that are abused.

Medical Imaging

Up to a third of a medical center's revenue comes from medical imaging performed by radiologists and cardiologists. These are tests, such as CT-scans, chest-X-rays, and coronary radionucleotide imaging studies.

Medical imaging is a bigger cost to the system than laboratory tests (i.e. blood work).[82] Lab tests comprise 11% of the Medicare expenditures and imaging studies make up 17%, according to a recent study.

CT-scans are probably the most profitable for a hospital. MRI imaging for back pain is another big waste of money.

A recent report in JAMA listed the most overused medical treatments, and imaging studies dominated the list. [83] Specifically, the following studies are the biggest wastes of money and sources of radiation damage to the patient:

Transesophageal echocardiography: This complex procedure requires the patient to be sedated in an operating room as an endoscope of pushed down the esophagus in order to get better ultrasound images of the heart. However,

---

[82] Litkowski P, et al. "Curbing the Urge to Image" *The Am. Journ. Med.*, October 2016. Vol. 129, Issue 10, 1131 - 1135

[83] Morgan D, et al. 2017 "Update on Medical Overuse: A Systematic Review" *JAMA Intern Med.* 2018;178(1):110-115

normal handheld ultrasound studies can be just as useful in most cases.

Computed tomography (i.e. CT-scan) pulmonary angiography: If a patient is suspected of having a life-threatening blood clot that broke off from a leg vessel and traveled to the lungs, this time-consuming test has gained popularity in diagnosing. It not only delivers a large amount of radiation, but is inconclusive many times. Of note, most patients receiving CT-scans are vulnerable, in distress, and intimidated by the emergency room setting, woefully unable to question the need or a study.

Computed tomography in any patients with respiratory symptoms: If a patient has a cough or is suspected of having pneumonia, regular chest X-rays will suffice. Chest CT-scans are dangerous, costly, and find false positives that lead to unnecessary biopsies.

Carotid artery ultrasonography and stenting: Most people have some amount of atherosclerosis in the arteries after a certain age. Placing an ultrasound on the neck of a patient without symptoms of stroke to look at the carotids leads to unnecessary coronary stenting or surgical procedure (i.e. carotid endarterectomy). Those procedures have a significant risk of stroke as the devices dislodge plaque that flows to the brain. The cardiologists performing these imaging studies then refer to themselves to do the stenting, which is an unethical conflict of interest.

Cardiac imaging: There are numerous imaging studies that the typical heart patient undergoes. Most of them are unnecessary for diagnosis and do not improve outcomes.

Over the last decade, a very concerning scam has blossomed. It is the use of a CT-scanner, which delivers huge amounts of radiation, to study the coronary arteries of the heart to look for blockades. What the studies find in almost everyone are white calcifications. Then, the same cardiologists that prescribed the expensive CT-scan refer the patients to their own cardiac cath-labs to undergo stenting.

Other overused cardiology tests include stress imaging studies. The patient receives intravenous injections of radioactive markers, which are damaging to the kidneys and risk causing cancer. But the use of these studies on any patient other than high-risk groups is a waste of time and harmful to the patient.

Mammograms: The use of mammograms to detect breast cancer has been in the news over the last several years. The proper frequency of the test is now controversial. The American Cancer Society advises mammograms for women aged 40 to 44 on an induvial-choice basis. For those aged 45 to 54, a yearly mammogram is advised, and for those 55 and, every other year. However, the U.S. Preventive Services Task Force (USPSTF) recommends mammograms for women starting at 50, not 45, and every two years up to age 74, and then no screening at all after age 74. They say that beginning screening before the age of 50 should be an individual decision based on your personal needs and risks.[84]

---

[84] All of these guidelines are pretty much useless, because the individual risk factors for each patient overrides broad population studies. For example, women who have a family history or have certain genetic mutation should be more aggressive than others.

Laboratory Tests

Most people would guess that lab tests (i.e. *in vitro* diagnostics done on blood taken from the patient) make the most money for the hospital. That used to be the case, but Medicare got wise and cut reimbursement rates.

Now, the radiology lobbyists have gained the upper hand and the radiologists make more money for the hospitals with medical imaging. Nevertheless, lab tests are still 10% or more of a given hospital's revenue. That means they are overutilized in many cases.

Overused Surgical Procedures

Patients who need some sort of surgery or procedure make more money for the hospital than a pure medical admission to treat pneumonia, for example. So, of course, there exists the big problem of doctors making false diagnoses in order to treat them with unnecessary procedures.

As a surgeon who has trained for periods of time with all of the sub-specialties, such as cardiac, vascular, transplant, and plastic surgery, I can tell you that many of the cases performed in America are unnecessary. I only know this now, decades later, after I got older and wiser.

Unwittingly, I participated in scams that harmed patients. It makes me sick to think now that, as a naïve intern, I was helping one of the busiest cardiac surgery teams in South Florida, and then in New York the next year, do coronary artery bypass procedures. Most of the patients did not benefit from a reduced chance of heart attack after the surgery, but all of them suffered serious harm from the heart bypass machine, vein harvesting, etc.

I have witnessed so many atrocities at the hands of incompetent surgeons motivated by the wrong factors that I actually wrote a screenplay (i.e. a "treatment") for a medical drama. I never got around to making a movie or TV show. This book will have to suffice.

It should be noted that most of the surgeons operating at respectable medical centers are very qualified. They are the best of the best, like the astronauts in the 1960's or elite military teams. But like so many professions, medicine and surgery does not weed out the bad ones. The unsafe surgeons find a home somewhere. Even when the surgeons are very competent, greed can cause them to harm patients, as I saw during my surgery training days.

Orthopedic and Spine Procedures

Some of the most common ailments are painful shoulders, hips, knees, and backs. The pain from these orthopedic injuries is debilitating. As a result, the patients demand surgery and third party payers cover them, regardless of efficacy. The squeaky wheel gets the grease.

It is very frustrating for me to hear men on the golf course, for example, talking about their ailments and surgeries. It is unethical for me to volunteer my advice, but I wish I could.

Any successful orthopedic surgeon is making 10-times or more than that of an internist or family doctor. The hospitals receive a separate facility fee for the operating rooms. As a result, over the last several decades, the number of orthopedic surgeries has exploded.

Knee and hip replacement surgeries are true modern miracles. I would not deter any patient with arthritis from having one. Although I do encourage second opinions to make sure that one truly has a need for an implant.

There are numerous smaller procedures that usually accompany these big surgeries. Many of them are unnecessary.

Knee scoping (i.e. arthroscopy) is a procedure done on many young people with sports injuries. In addition to making a diagnosis, the theory is that, by cleaning out loose cartilage, arthroscopy benefits the patient. A greedy surgeon can do many cases a day. Well, a large study showed that knee scoping was utterly ineffective.[85]

Injecting the knee joint with slippery hyaluronic acid compounds to reduce the friction of the bone-on-bone contact can be beneficial for early arthritis. Therefore, Medicare and insurance pays for it. As a result, knee injections have become abused by orthopedic surgery centers. When a patient clearly needs an implant, they will waste time and money with a series of injections.

Shoulder surgery is something that nobody should undergo unless they have given their injury six-months to heal. The vast majority of "torn rotator cuffs" heal on their own. Moreover, the surgeries are often ineffective.

---

[85] Mounsey A, et al. "Arthroscopic surgery for knee osteoarthritis? Just say no" *J Fam Pract*. 2009 Mar; 58(3): 143–145

Spine surgery for back pain is a scam, pure and simple. There is no other way of putting it. The surgeries rarely alleviate pain. Large clinical trials have shown that outcomes are no better after surgery than if the patient did not undergo surgery.

Investigative journalist Cathryn Ramin detailed this scam in her book.[86] Spine surgery is a $100 Billion industry. Spine fusion surgery (i.e. where metal screws and plates are used to fuse together adjacent vertebrae) works only 35% of the time. Despite the data, spine fusion cases performed annually have increased 600% between 1993 and 2011 (from 61,000 to 465,000). In a poll of spine surgeons, 99% would not undergo spine fusion surgery themselves.

If you undergo an MRI of the spine and are told that you have a herniated disc, or some other deformity needing surgery, be very skeptical. Almost everyone has an abnormality in their spine and they are walking around just fine. Even if the herniated disc that you might have is causing the back pain, it will be dissolved and eaten up by your body's immune cells over six-months or so and you will be just as well off as if you had undergone surgery. Only if you have numbness in the extremities should you consider back surgery.

If you suffer a sudden back pain from bending over the wrong way, take an aspirin or NSAID to reduce the inflammation. Then, find an overhead bar and dangle from it for a few seconds. Inversion tables are good too. These decompress the spine.

---

[86] Ramin C. "Crooked: Outwitting the Back Pain Industry and Getting on the Road to Recovery" Harper 2017

Coronary Stents and CABG Surgery

I am one of the leading experts on stenting, having followed the clinical data for decades. When I began my Wall Street career, I was assigned to write the very first report on drug-coated coronary stents (now called "drug eluting" stents).[87]

Stents are small metal coils that are positioned inside a coronary artery blockage to help get blood flowing to the heart muscle. The drug coatings help prevent the arterial wall from growing back and reforming a blockage (i.e. restenosis).

Well, soon after Johnson & Johnson got the first stent approved in 2001, doctors started to notice strange things happening to the vessels. They were ballooning out, forming aneurysms. Those aneurysms can form deadly blood clots leading to heart attacks. What was causing this new phenomenon was the polymer coating the stent, which was acting as a foreign body irritant. The inflammatory process weakens the arteries.

But these safety signals did not deter the aggressive interventional cardiologists (i.e. the cardiology mafia), who were drunk with power. Their new lucrative procedures were putting the open-heart surgeons out of business. They were the new kings of the hospitals, having never undergone the strenuous surgery training.

We now have nearly two-decades of real-world data on coronary stenting. Multiple studies show that they do not reduce the chance of heart attack or death. They do not even reduce chest pain (i.e. angina).

In 2007, the large trial known as COURAGE found no benefit from stenting in the form of reduction in

---

[87] Greer SE, Hopkins B. "They're Here! Radiation, Drug-Coated Stents, and Other Anti-Restenosis Therapies" Credit-Suisse First Boston research. November 7, 2000.

cardiovascular adverse events or death.[88] Stents did not even treat stable angina. The chest pain returned. Then, in 2017, a paper in Lancet also showed that stents did not reduce angina, which many saw as the last nail in the coffin for stenting.[89]

But stents do cause tremendous morbidity. Because of the aneurysms caused by the coatings and risk of clotting and heart attack, patients with stents have to take expensive blood thinners for life. As mentioned above, these blood thinners, such as Xarelto and Eliquis, are some of the biggest blockbuster drugs on the market.

Also, blood thinners do not come without life-threatening deadly risk. They cause serious bleeding into the brain or GI tract. They limit the physical activity of the patient. The cardiologists created a problem with stenting that now has to be treated by drugs. This violates the doctrine of "First, do no harm"

As these adverse events from stents have become known, stenting started to decline in practice. So, many cardiologists bought their own CT-scanners to perform cancer-causing scans of the heart. When a white spot of calcium shows up, the doctors refer to themselves for the stenting. No other specialty self-refers like this.

Despite no supporting data, coronary calcium screening is a common test performed. President 43, George W. Bush, a healthy man who exercises, was harmed by a group of Texas doctors who ordered one of these scans during an "executive physical". Of course, it showed some calcium in his coronaries, as almost everyone has, and he

---

[88] Boden W, et al. "Optimal Medical Therapy with or without PCI for Stable Coronary Disease" *N Engl J Med.* 2007, Apr 12;356(15):1503-16

[89] Brown D, et al. "Last nail in the coffin for PCI in stable angina?" *Lancet.* Volume 391, ISSUE 10115, P3-4, January 06, 2018

underwent coronary stenting, despite having no chest pain. He has since been quoted as complaining about how easily he bleeds now.

President Bush needed a medical advocate. Instead, he blindly listened to the doctors (the same way that he was misled into the Iraq and Afghanistan wars, and poorly handled the financial crisis, but I digress).

Before stenting, highly morbid open-heart surgery (i.e. coronary artery bypass graft surgery, or CABG) was the overused procedure of the day. But like stenting, study after study has shown CABG to be of little benefit.[90]

Meanwhile, the surgery harms the brain (i.e. "pump brain")[91] The leg vein harvesting is also painful and ugly. Sternal infections are a common problem too. Yet plenty of people still undergo needless CABG. American hero Neil Armstrong, who defied death as a test pilot and astronaut, was killed by CABG.[92]

The decision of whether or not to undergo stenting or CABG is a complex one that a non-biased medical advocate can assist with greatly. The doctors recommending the procedures are almost always too biased to be trustworthy.

---

[90] Adelborg K, et al. "Thirty-Year Mortality After Coronary Artery Bypass Graft SurgeryA Danish Nationwide Population-Based Cohort Study" *Circulation*. Vol. 10, No. 5. May, 2017

[91] Newman M, et al. "Longitudinal Assessment of Neurocognitive Function after Coronary-Artery Bypass Surgery" *N Engl J Med* 2001; 344:395-402

[92] Kolata G. "Neil Armstrong Died After Heart Surgery. That May Have Been Avoidable." *New York Times*. July 25, 2019. https://www.nytimes.com/2019/07/25/health/neil-armstrong-heart-surgery.html

The ICU

In the 1950s, Austrian-born, Yale and Penn-trained, anesthesiologist Peter Safar began working in the laboratory on the concept that saving the brain from death by maintaining blood flow was of paramount importance. He had already pioneered Cardiopulmonary Resuscitation (CPR).

The critically-ill had been dying from respiratory distress. In 1958, he is credited with forming the first Intensive Care Unit (ICU). He sedated critically ill patients in order to allow them to be intubated and placed on ventilators.

But the invention of the ICU has opened a Pandora's Box. While the benefits of modern ICU care have been unquestionable, the harms are lesser known.

Most of the important procedures in the ICU have never been validated by clinical trials. Doctors experiment *ad hoc* on ways to ventilate, provide vasoconstricting drugs, monitor blood pressure with special catheters going inside the heart (Swan-Ganz catheters), monitor heart dysrhythmias, and fight hypovolemic shock or bacterial sepsis shock.

Trust me when I tell you that very few doctors have a clue what they are doing in the ICU. The doctors in charge are usually still in training. Moreover, as I mentioned, there lacks good data to support the techniques used. It is dogma.

The Swan-Ganz catheter, for example, which goes through the right atrium of the heart into the pulmonary artery going to the lungs, has been a mainstay of the ICU. It provides an overload of data that serve to confuse and distract doctors, for the most part.

A 2013 New England Journal of Medicine review stated[93]:

> "Although pulmonary -artery catheterization had historically been the standard of care for all critically ill patients, data from randomized, controlled trials have shown that it offers no clear benefits to patients with septic shock,[94] acute respiratory distress syndrome,[95] or acute decompensated heart failure.[96] Similarly, pulmonary-artery catheterization offers no clear benefits in the routine treatment of patients undergoing high-risk surgery. In such populations, cardiac function and volume status should instead be assessed through noninvasive means when possible, including physical examination, measurement of B-type natriuretic peptide levels, echocardiography, measurement of variations in pulse pressure during respiration, and sonographic assessment of the diameter of the inferior vena cava

---

[93] Kelly C, Rabbani L. "Pulmonary-Artery Catheterization" *N Engl J Med* 2013;369:25

[94] Richard C, Warszawski J, Anguel N, et al. "Early use of the pulmonary artery catheter and outcomes in patients with shock and acute respiratory distress syndrome: a randomized controlled trial" *JAMA* 2003;290:2713-2720

[95] "The National Heart, Lung, and Blood Institute Acute Respiratory Distress Syndrome (ARDS) Clinical Trials Network. Pulmonary-artery versus central venous catheter to guide treatment of acute lung injury" *N Engl J Med* 2006;354:2213-2224

[96] Binanay C, Califf RM, Hasselblad V, et al. "Evaluation study of congestive heart failure and pulmonary artery catheterization effectiveness: the ESCAPE trial" *JAMA* 2005;294:1625-1633

during respiration. In patients with acute respiratory distress syndrome, treatment determined on the basis of central venous pressure, which can be obtained with a simple central venous catheter, yields outcomes equivalent to those of treatment determined on the basis of pulmonary-capillary wedge pressure." [97]

Yet, despite these studies showing the futility of this expensive and dangerous procedure, Swan-Ganz catheters are still commonly used in American ICUs. As long as Medicare and insurance will pay hospitals, they will be used.

Regarding the routine use of sedation and ventilation, there are no trials to show that this saves lives. Doctors do not even have good guidelines as to when to initiate the procedure. In most cases, it is a completely subjective decision by the doctor.

A 2012 medical journal reported[98]:

"Critically ill patients are routinely provided analgesia and sedation to prevent pain and anxiety, permit invasive procedures, reduce stress and oxygen consumption, and improve synchrony with mechanical ventilation. Regional

---

[97] Richard C, Warszawski J, Anguel N, et al. "Early use of the pulmonary artery catheter and outcomes in patients with shock and acute respiratory distress syndrome: a randomized controlled trial" *JAMA* 2003;290:2713-2720

[98] Hughes C, et al. "Sedation in the intensive care setting" *Clin Pharmacol.* 2012; 4:53–63

preferences, patient history, institutional bias, and individual patient and practitioner variability, however, create a wide discrepancy in the approach to sedation of critically ill patients. Untreated pain and agitation increase the sympathetic stress response, potentially leading to negative acute and long-term consequences. Oversedation, however, occurs commonly and is associated with worse clinical outcomes, including longer time on mechanical ventilation, prolonged stay in the intensive care unit, and increased brain dysfunction (delirium and coma). Modifying sedation delivery by incorporating analgesia and sedation protocols, targeted arousal goals, daily interruption of sedation, linked spontaneous awakening and breathing trials, and early mobilization of patients have all been associated with improvements in patient outcomes and should be incorporated into the clinical management of critically ill patients. To improve outcomes, including time on mechanical ventilation and development of acute brain dysfunction, conventional sedation paradigms should be altered by providing necessary analgesia, incorporating propofol or dexmedetomidine to reach arousal targets, and reducing benzodiazepine exposure."

A very concerning trend sweeping the country is for hospitals to build fancy new buildings in which all of the hospital rooms can be converted into ICUs. See if you can guess what is motivating this. Are there suddenly more critically ill patients, or do ICU's make more money for the hospital?

Bingo. The latter is the correct answer. An ICU patient allows the hospital bill for much more than a simpler admission. As I mentioned previously, bloated inefficient hospitals are losing money despite seeing increases in revenue. They only know how to do one thing, which is to increase revenue by any means possible. They will never cut expenses until they are forced to do so.

You probably know somebody who was recently diagnosed with pneumonia. That is a vague and somewhat arbitrary diagnosis being made more and more because it justifies the ICU designation and billing codes.

Silos of Specialists Not Communicating With One Another

Another reason that there are so many unnecessary or redundant tests ordered, and so many medical mistakes made, is that the American healthcare system is rewarded for operating within insulated silos. Anyone who has had even just a basic annual physical knows that they get bounced around from one office to another. For the seriously ill, the problem is a true crisis.

Gone are the days when you had a true primary care doctor acting as the quarterback or central hub for your care. The corrupt American reimbursement system has been rigged to pay the specialists far more than the primary care doctor. Few want to go into primary care or family medicine. For those who still do, they have now been replaced by their medical centers with floating hospitalists acting much like the on-call resident in training.

The problems with the new hospitalist system are manifold. For starters, there is a different hospitalist every shift. This creates a lack of continuity of care. They can read notes in the hospital records to get up to speed, but that is a far cry from the care delivered by one single primary care doctor who has known you for years and knows every detail of your current hospitalization. Then, most hospitalists are not exactly the cream of the crop, to say the least. It is a crummy job and they are doing it for a reason. But even if they are very good doctors, the current system is not conducive for communication.

The typical hospital care for a patient will start with an emergency room doctor making a diagnosis. Then, some sort of specialist doctor is brought in to make the admission. Astonishingly, your primary care doctor is often not alerted at all. Depending on the type of specialist, you might rarely even see the doctor who is supposed to be in charge of your care.

The typical patient in a hospital is too sick and scared to ask the names of the various people walking in with blue scrubs or white coats. The new trend in American medicine is to recognize all forms of hospital staff as equal "providers", just as if they were MDs, and patients have no way of knowing what level of training a particular caregiver has.

Probably the most important service that we offer as a medical advocate is to keep track of who is treating you and why. Then, we make sure that the doctors who need to know your status know.

American Healthcare Ignores Preventive Care

Another way that the American healthcare system can harm you is by failing to address the reasons that you get sick in the first place. There are few financial incentives for preventive care.

I have a relative in the Midwest who is obese. I saw that it was causing a sequela of ailments and a serious deterioration in quality of life. So, I tried my best to find some sort of professional medical-center-level of dietary coaching. To make a long story short, none existed.

The most common diseases in the United States are not what you would think. They are not heart disease or cancer. Those are just sequela (i.e. consequences of) other diseases, such as food, alcohol, and tobacco addictions, or the glorification of violence. Not only are those true causations not treated by formal American healthcare, but they are actually promoted by the nation as a whole.

The food, alcohol, tobacco, film, and video game industries make too much money for any government agency to crack down on them. One sees the confluence of these sleazy industries at sporting events, where violence and alcohol are the main events. Our culture and economy revolve around disease, much as it does with constant costly military conflicts.

The aforementioned industries of disease fit in perfectly with the $3.6 Trillion American healthcare industry scam. They are synergistic. That is why you see advertisements at ballgames for medical centers and endorsements from medical societies for certain foods that are not healthy at all.

If everyone ate healthily, drank alcohol in moderation, never smoked, and avoided risky violence, the rates of diabetes, arthritis, heart disease, cancer, and homicide would plummet, putting hospitals out of business. Instead, America has a majority of the population that strives to become sick, and drugs or medical devices are the cures.

American Healthcare Emphasizes Drugs and Devices

Hospitals only care for you when you are sick. They have no need for healthy people. Preventive care is not on their radar.

Sure, hospitals have plenty of social awareness campaigns on preventive medicine, but it is all mostly lip-service. Charity marathons and bike races do not prevent cancer. They only serve as huge public relations stunts for the nearby cancer center.

Indeed, entire industries of non-profits pretending to promote health exist. Follow the money. Look at the "901" forms filed by the non-profits and see the million-dollar salaries earned by those do-gooders. Cancer research receives a small fraction of the donations in many cases.

Pink-ribbon month in October, promoted by the NFL, for example, only helps the Komen Foundation scam. Indeed, the founder and CEO, Susan Goodman, was ousted after scandal. The largest spending category for the foundations is for self-promotional pink-ribbon campaigns. A small percentage (5%) goes toward treating cancer. Twice as much (11%) goes toward executive salaries.

Other preventive medicine services offered by hospitals are not promoted much because the hospitals receive little reimbursement for them. They have mostly focused on reducing stress, increasing exercise, improving diet, and stopping smoking for their own employees. But the typical patient admitted and then discharged for some ailment caused by obesity, for example, is not given basic instructions on how to attend clinics on diet, for example. Even obvious killer habits, such as smoking, are ignored.

Once you become sick and are admitted to the hospital, the doctors will deliver numerous therapies using expensive drugs and medical devices. That keeps them in business. Far too often, these therapies simply do not work and end up harming the patient.

Our medical advocacy service makes sure that the patient truly needs the therapies being recommended. When they are appropriate, we make sure that you know the true risks and benefits.

"Do Not Resuscitate" Interpreted as License to Euthanize

Patients are often asked by the hospital whether they wish to be placed on a ventilator should they become comatose or whether they would like to have "Do Not Resuscitate", or DNR, orders. It seems like a rational thing to do, to be on DNR status. Who would want to be in a vegetative coma state on a ventilator? But in reality, a DNR order on a patient immediately changes the care given. It is interpreted as "Do Not Treat", and the patient might as well be in a hospice home preparing to die.

In my experience, DNR orders are often put in place by family members overwhelmed by a sick parent. Sometimes, the family member simply does not want the burden of caring for the elder relative. In other instances, the family member has been misled by the hospital about DNR.

The most dramatic results from our medical advocacy are seen in the lone elderly sick patient. Their lack of family support at the bedside often makes them give up hope. They believe that death is imminent, when in many cases that is not true.

Our medical advocacy service strongly recommends that DNR orders not be used unless the patient is truly terminal. In that case, they should be in a hospice program and not a hospital. There should not be this pseudo-hospice within hospitals known as DNR.

Hospitals are powerful tools and should be used to prolong life, regardless of patient age. There is no "duty to die" If someone has a functioning brain and is not in agonizing pain, they deserve a shot at life.

American Healthcare Violates Your Privacy

One of the worst consequences of the Affordable Care Act, or Obamacare, was the mandated implementation of electronic medical records (EMR) by hospitals. It created a new industry where EMR companies exploit the pseudo-government incompetent nature of hospitals and price gouge them for tens of millions of dollars for EMR software that is full of glitches.

Patients are now complaining that doctors spend most of their time staring at laptops entering notes rather than looking at them. A new hospital job called transcriptionist has arisen, whereby people follow the doctor from exam room to exam room transcribing what the doctor says.

But worse than the waste and inefficiency of EMR is the violation of privacy. Your most sensitive private information found in your medical records is now vulnerable and likely to be gathered by third-parties and used for profit. This is the real reason why a provision to mandate EMR was stuffed into the Obamacare bill that few people read, and why Newt Gingrich became such an advocate of EMR.

Various industries would love to know the details about you found in your medical records in order to target you for marketing. Sick people spend a lot of money on drugs and other healthcare products and services. "Efficiency" and "patient safety" were just canards used to push through EMR.

We live in an age of what has been dubbed *Surveillance Capitalism.*[99] It is an economy where you are the product. All of your personal information revealed through your Internet searches and social media posts are used to sell to other companies that want to focus their marketing campaigns.

Surveillance Capitalism probably started with Google. Then, after Google become the second largest company in the world, others started to copy the business model. Now, car companies are selling your driving data. Robot vacuum cleaners are making digital floor plan maps of your home and uploading them. Smart-home devices, such Amazon's *Alexa,* are recording your voice and transcribing it into written documents. Google-owned *Nest* thermostats even have hidden speakers that no one was told about, which listens in on you and transcribes forever what you say. Amazon's *Ring* video doorbells sell your home videos to police, and god knows who else. Finally, of course, your smart phone is nothing but an eavesdropping spy gadget.

Google (now called Alphabet) and Amazon have large divisions that sell cloud computing storage to the

---

[99] Zuboff S. "The Age of Surveillance Capitalism" PublicAffairs, Hachette Book Group. 2019.

CIA, military, and private industry. Guess what. They are vying for contracts with various medical centers to store your electronic medical records.[100] What could go wrong?

The pattern of abuse by all of these Big Tech companies is to first egregiously steal and sell your personal data. Then, when the feckless government catches them, the companies apologize, promise to not do it again, and get a slap on the wrist. I would be shocked if that does not happen in the near future with EMR.

In fact, this has been going on for decades and the Supreme Court ruled it was legal in *Sorrell v. IMS Health Inc.*, 564 U.S. 552 (2011). The State of Vermont passed a law making it illegal for IMS Health to collect the prescribing data from doctors' office and sell it to marketers. But the court ruled that it was a violation of the First Amendment. Say what?

There is a federal law called the Health Insurance Portability and Accountability Act (HIPAA) that was passed under the Clinton administration to supposedly secure your medical information. Slowly, the industry lobbyists have chipped away at it, watering it down to the point where our Supreme Court thwarts state efforts to protect your sensitive health records.

Aside from official medical records, Big Tech is collecting your medical data from other sources. Pharmacy chains and credit card companies sell the data on your purchases.

And those genetic tests advertised on TV, such as Google-owned *23andMe*, are the worst ideas ever. First,

---

[100] Evans M. "Google, Amazon and Microsoft in Battle to Store Health Data in the Cloud." *Wall Street Journal.* September 10, 2019.

they do not predict diseases as promised.[101] The FDA took *23andMe* off the market for false advertising. Then, the DNA collected is the Holy Grail for surveillance capitalism companies. Already, we know enough about the human genome to tell the race, sex, and ethnicity of a person from their DNA. Very soon, we will indeed be able to predict disease, which will mean that the medical companies can start bombarding you with ads before you are even sick.

Nursing Homes are Often as Bad as You Fear

Two of my main areas of treatment in my Quality of Life Clinic medical practice are geriatrics and chronic wounds. I got into this field back in my surgery residency days at NYU when I designed a multi-center clinical trial testing a new type of chronic wound treatment called negative pressure therapy.[102] I was awarded two federal research grants from the Veterans Affairs, and also worked with an NIH-funded wing of Bellevue Hospital for help with statistical analysis.[103]

In order to enroll patients who met the protocol requirements, I had to venture out into the community and visit long-term care "nursing homes" Very few doctors leave the hospital or office and travel to the patient. The American healthcare machine does not reward house calls with payments.

Nursing homes usually have one part-time doctor overseeing care. But most nursing homes are just fancy

---

[101] Klitzman R, Greer SE. "The 23andMe home genetics test kit controversy." *The Healthcare Channel*. December 19, 2013

[102] Greer SE: "Whither Subatmospheric Pressure Dressing? Editorial" *Ann Plast Surg,* 45(3):332-4, 2000 (see my *curriculum vitae* at the end of the book for the entire list)

[103] See me *curriculum vitae* at the end of this book

apartments with services to help with food and care. They are not hospitals. They are also regulated less than hospitals.

As a result, the quality of care at nursing homes ranges widely from good to horrific. Basic orders left by a doctor for how to change a wound dressing, for example, often go ignored or carried out improperly.

In 1998, I quickly spotted this unmet clinical need and pioneered the concept of the traveling wound doctor. There are now several national companies doing this, but I was the first.

Every problem with American healthcare that I have previously listed is amplified in the outpatient long-term care setting. It is the Wild West.

There is a totally different mindset to patient care in the nursing home. Caregivers and children of patients often have given up and are treating the patient as if they are terminally ill and in hospice. Sometimes, that is appropriate, but far too often, it is not right. I mentioned before about the DNR status being misinterpreted as Do Not Treat.

Elderly patients with dementia from Alzheimer's or other degenerative diseases are true challenges for everyone. Many require antipsychotic medications to sedate them. But many patients who should not be on these medications are receiving them.

One thing I do is assess the list of medications my patients are on and decide if any should be stopped. Antipsychotics, for example, lead to other diseases, such as diabetes, as "side effects" In the FDA label is a black box warning that they increase the chance of death.

Another common problem I see in nursing homes is malnutrition. Again, the patients with dementia are difficult to feed. They develop low albumin levels and this leads to chronic wounds that do not heal. But in most cases, liquid protein supplements work well. I am surprised at how many geriatric doctors overlook nutritional status.

When it comes time for families to choose a nursing home, the cost is the main issue. But other than that, families have little ability to judge based on the care given. Our medical advocacy service can be of great assistance there. It takes an insider to know what is going on.

Once you or your loved one is placed into a nursing home, our service will send staff by routinely to provide oversight and look out for red flags. For example, if the patient is immobile and at risk for bed sores, we will recommend a special mattress be added to the care regime. If excessive unnecessary medications are being prescribe, we will make recommendations to the doctor in charge.

Chapter 8. The Real Risks

I mentioned before that I was truly naïve as a surgery resident about the scams taking place in the cardiac surgery teams for which I worked. But there is something else about which I cannot plead ignorance. It is the process of obtaining written consent from the patient before surgery.

It is the job of the lowest person on the surgery totem pole to frantically run around during clinic sessions to do rushed history and physicals (H&P). Part of the process, usually done by the first-year intern, is explaining to the patient the risks of the procedure.

In reality, doctors make up these statistics. The usual song and dance is that there is only a "one-percent chance of infection", etc. In fact, risks to surgical and other procedures are often many times greater than what doctors want to admit or disclose to the patient.[104]

Many adverse events are not even considered as risks from the procedure. If an interventional cardiology procedure is found many days later to have caused a mild stroke, the cardiologists do not admit to it, for example.

It is not just surgical risks that are glossed over by the doctors. Many drugs, particularly chemotherapy drugs, are so toxic that they kill a large percentage of patients. Despite those adverse events, the official medical journal publications of the trial data often describe the drugs as "generally well tolerated"

---

[104] Bismark M, Gawande A, et al. "Legal Disputes over Duties to Disclose Treatment Risks to Patients: A Review of Negligence Claims and Complaints in Australia" *PLoS Medicine*, 2012; 9 (8)

An essay from Harvard researchers detailed this problem of researchers failing to inform doctors of the true risks of drugs:[105]

>""Safe and effective." "Manageable toxicities." "Generally well tolerated." Medical journal articles, often in the field of oncology but increasingly in other specialties as well, propagate such reassuring characterizations of new therapies. But these seemingly straightforward descriptions belie patients' complex and varied experiences. In one study comparing two treatment regimens in patients with metastatic colorectal cancer, adverse events led to discontinuation of chemotherapy in 39% of patients in one treatment group and 27% in the other. In total, 13 people died from an adverse event. The investigators concluded that "treatment was well tolerated." In a study of 50 patients with advanced Merkel cell carcinoma, 28% of participants had a grade 3 or 4 treatment-related adverse event, which led to discontinuation of treatment in 14%; one of these events was a death. The therapy was reported to have "a generally manageable safety profile." Similar examples are everywhere....
>
>Improving physicians' communication with patients about

---

[105] Sacks C. *et al*. "Talking about Toxicity — "What We've Got Here Is a Failure to Communicate"" *NEJM*. 381;15. October 10, 2019

possible risks and benefits of treatments has long been recognized as a critical priority. But perhaps a necessary first step is for investigators to communicate with clinicians openly and specifically about the toxic effects of treatment."

Ironically, this essay was published in the hypocritical *New England Journal of Medicine*, which is the venue for every large industry-funded drug trial publication for a new chemotherapy drug. Do the editors think that, by publishing this essay, they are absolved? Also, the authors work for the Harvard company of doctors known as Partners.org, which is perhaps the biggest offender of fee-for-service overutilization of services in the country.

One service of our medical advocate service is to give you unbiased accurate assessments of risk. Even very common drugs, such as aspirin, have huge risks of deadly adverse events.

Chapter 9. The Red Flag Specialties

Again, I emphasize that the vast majority of medical doctors and other healthcare providers are honest, well-intentioned, adequately-trained, people. But the few doctors in the system who tend to order the most unnecessary tests and procedures are responsible for an inordinate share of the problem. Who are these doctors and how can you be on guard?

Oncology

I have long told people within my inner circle, "You don't want to get cancer.", and I have not been referring to the actual diseases of cancer. I have been cynically warning about the entire oncology industry that has become corrupted to the core.

Financial conflicts-of-interest have metastasized to all stages of the cancer treatment process. This financial tumor has flourished in a culture of virtually no oversight. Politicians and the regulatory bodies they control do not want to be smeared as obstructionists to cancer care.

Oncologists and drug companies have evaded the normal immune response of the government oversight bodies, just like real cancer tumors do. The following are some of the tactics they use.

False Diagnoses of "Cancer"

The first step for cancer patients is being told that they have been diagnosed with cancer. Well, not all diagnoses are objective and accurate. Some diagnoses are completely bogus.

"Breast cancer", for example, is a diagnosis that is often a fake diagnosis. "Stage 0", or low risk ductal carcinoma in situ (DCIS), "breast cancer" is not real cancer. It is only a subjective finding of "abnormal cells" found on biopsy.[106] Yet millions of young women have been treated as if they have deadly breast cancer, undergoing chemotherapy and mastectomy.

A growing trend is for women without genetic risk factors for breast cancer, such as the various BRCA gene mutations, voluntarily opting to have both breasts removed out of fear of possible future breast cancer.[107] Celebrities, such as Angelina Jolie, set the trend.

"Thyroid cancer" is another disease on the rise due to false diagnoses.[108] Small papillary thyroid nodules are simply abnormal looking cells. New technologies are getting too sensitive and picking up things that would have been ignored in previous years.

Prostate cancer is a very controversial diagnosis. Most cases diagnosed are slow-growing and may never kill the patient. The decision on how to treat prostate cancer must be tailored to each patient based on risk factors.

---

[106] Elmore J, et al. "Overdiagnosis in Breast Cancer Screening: Time to Tackle an Underappreciated Harm" *Ann Intern Med.* 2012 Apr 3; 156(7): 536–537. https://thehcc.tv November, 2013.

[107] Winchester D, Greer SE. "Increasing rates of double mastectomies in early stage breast cancer" The Healthcare Channel. November 22, 2013

[108] Jegerlehner S, et al. "Overdiagnosis and overtreatment of thyroid cancer: A population-based temporal trend study" *PLoS One.* 2017; 12(6): e0179387.

The Chemotherapy Mark-Up

A long time ago, Medicare tried to do a good thing and cut the cost of cancer care. It encouraged outpatient oncology offices to administer chemotherapy by allowing those offices to sell the chemotherapy drugs at a mark-up of about 6%. This profit margin on drugs now comprises the majority of revenue for an oncology office. It has resulted in one of the biggest scams in American medicine.

The more expensive the drug, the more revenue the oncology office makes. Therefore, it is of no surprise that cancer drugs now cost several hundreds of thousand dollars per patient. New cell-based therapies are breaking through the million-dollar barrier.[109]

Not only do these costly chemo bills hurt the patient in co-pays and out-of-pocket costs, and make cancer care impossible for the uninsured, but they also discourage the use of more effective drugs if they are cheaper.

No cancer patient can possibly navigate this minefield. It is not like shopping for a car. First, the drug prices are not disclosed. Secondly, the patients lack the medical knowledge to know which drugs should or should not be used. Our medical advocacy service helps with this.

---

[109] Szabo L. "Cascade of Costs Could Push New Gene Therapy Above $1 Million Per Patient" *Kaiser Health News* website. October 17, 2017. https://khn.org/news/cascade-of-costs-could-push-new-gene-therapy-above-1-million-per-patient/

Unproven Radiation Therapy

In medical school, I was thinking of going into otolaryngology (ENT), mostly for the reconstructive surgery aspect of the profession. I ended up pursuing pure plastic surgery.

Both specialties deal with surgical reconstruction after tumors are removed. After surgery, adjuvant radiation therapy is often delivered to the region. The theory is that the toxic radiation will kill more cancer cells than healthy cells. However, the long-term effects to the non-cancerous tissues are serious. The skin around the mastectomy or neck dissection sites is never the same.

But certainly, all of the morbidity from radiation therapy is worth it because the risks of progression of cancer are lowered. Right? Well, in most cases, there are no proper clinical trials to support the use of radiation therapy. It is pure dogma. Of course, radiation therapy makes a lot of money for the cancer centers.

Overused Cancer Therapies

All of what I just laid out above is not controversial. The cancer societies have recognized these problems. In a 2011 article[110], oncologist Thomas Smith, MD provided a list of overused cancer drugs, other therapies, and diagnostic tests.

One of the cancer dugs that earns the most revenue for the drug companies are a class known as white-cell-stimulating-factors, or colony-stimulating-factors. The drugs are best known as Neupogen and Neulasta, made by

---

[110] Smith T, et al. "Bending the Cost Curve in Cancer Care" *N Engl J Med.* 2011 May 26; 364(21): 2060–206

Amgen. They are growth factors that stimulate the bone marrow stem cells to reproduce and send into the bloodstream infection-fighting white blood cells (i.e. T and B cells). Smith's article singles them out as being over-prescribed.

Despite the official cancer societies, in the form of Smith's article, stating in the biggest medical journal, The New England Journal of Medicine, that Neupogen and Neulasta should be used less, guess what impact this had on real-world clinical practice. You guessed it—none.

Neulasta, the drug that replaced the original Neupogen, is still growing at 5%. It makes Amgen about $5 Billion in revenue each year.

The flip-side of the Neulasta coin is that the same guidelines by Smith also recommended that chemotherapy doses be reduced in order to prevent the need for Neulasta-type drugs in the first place (chemotherapy drugs are toxic to the bone marrow, requiring the offsetting stimulation by Neulasta). Well, those too have been ignored by the oncologists and hospitals. Chemotherapy is their bread and butter. Oncologists will prescribe them regardless of efficacy or harm to the patient.

Everything, in fact, listed in the Smith guidelines have been ignored. Cancer patients are still receiving unnecessary medical imaging studies to monitor the cancer when it is futile, and receiving unproven cocktails of drugs when cancers progress beyond hope. The cancer doctors are still being paid based on drug usage rather than patient outcome.

I interviewed Dr. Smith in 2011 for my Healthcare Channel.[111] At the time, I thought his paper would be a

---

[111] Smith T, Greer SE. "Bending the Cost Curve in Cancer Care" *The Healthcare Channel*. May 25, 2011.

paradigm changer. Boy oh boy, was I naïve. Medical literature that exposes risks or problems with popular money-making therapies rarely makes a dent in real-world application.

Alternative Medicine Quackery

Preying upon the desperate and scared, alternative medicine quacks are easily found when one is diagnosed with cancer. There seems to be is always "some guy" in Mexico supposedly saving lives with a miracle cure unavailable in the U.S.

Alarmingly, these scams are promoted by once-respected American doctors who get TV shows. Dr. Oz, for example, is the biggest quack there is, in my opinion, and he was formerly a respected New York heart surgeon.[112,113,114] He then became drunk with fame and had to stoop to appealing to the daytime TV masses with alternative medicine. You can thank Oprah Winfrey for starting this type of nonsense on her show, and then creating Dr. Oz.

---

[112] Abel J. "Study: less than half of Dr. Oz's recommendations are actually supported by evidence" *Consumer Affairs* website. No date listed. https://www.consumeraffairs.com/news/study-less-than-half-of-dr-ozs-recommendations-are-actually-supported-by-evidence-121914.html

[113] Tilburt J, et al. "The Case of Dr. Oz: Ethics, Evidence, and Does Professional Self-Regulation Work?" *AMA J Ethics.* 2017;19(2):199-206.

[114] Mutnick A. "Senators scold Dr. Oz for weight-loss scams" *USA Today* June 18, 2014.

Spine Surgery

While cancer doctors exploit the fear of death, spine surgeons exploit the desperation caused by back pain. I have already detailed these scams above.

The large Dartmouth studies on spine surgery known as the SPORT trials[115], as well as many others since, have shown time after time that spine fusion surgery rarely works to alleviate back pain. Tiger Woods is a great example. He underwent numerous back surgeries and never recovered from the pain.

I mentioned in the foreword how my mother went to a spine surgeon for pain and was scheduled to undergo spine surgery. She smartly got a second opinion. She needed knee surgery, not spine surgery.

Back pain is not a black and white diagnosis. It is very subjective. Always seek a second opinion on this.

Cardiology

I have previously mentioned the numerous medical imaging tests and procedures often performed needlessly by cardiologists. The fact is that the entire field of cardiology has not made much of an impact on heart disease.

It is true that deaths attributed to "heart disease" are lower now than they were several decades ago, but that is probably simply due to far fewer Americans smoking. Lipitor, CABG, or stents had little to do with it, as I have detailed in the pharmaceutical chapters.

---

[115] Weinstein J, et al. "Surgical vs Nonoperative Treatment for Lumbar Disk HerniationThe Spine Patient Outcomes Research Trial (SPORT): A Randomized Trial" *JAMA*. 2006;296(20):2441-2450

The NIH convened a panel of cardiologists to try and pinpoint why heart disease is on the decline.[116] The results were published in a report with no clear conclusion.

Also, the definition of "heart disease" used by the CDC, American Heart Association (AHA), and American College of Cardiology (ACC), is often clinically meaningless. For example, hypertension places someone into the "heart disease" basket of the population just as if they have had a heart attack or stroke. By arbitrarily lowering the threshold of what defines hypertension, the cardiology community gains more potential patients. The drug companies that fund the AHA and ACC can sell more blood pressure medications. Cardiologists want us to believe that half of America has heart disease.[117]

Our medical advocacy service offers advice to patients about which of the many pills they have been told to take are truly helpful. In many cases, the cholesterol lowering drugs, aspirin, and blood pressure medications are doing more harm than good.

Obviously, many Americans have genuine heart disease and need a cardiologist to manage their heart failure, monitor their blood clotting if they have atrial fibrillation or a heart valve, etc. But a huge portion of the population has been labeled with "heart disease" and told to take medications that do not help them.

The best way to improve your cardiology health is by not smoking, eating better food, and doing a modest

---

[116] Mensah G, et al. "Decline in Cardiovascular Mortality: Possible Causes and Implications" *Circ Res.* 2017 Jan 20; 120(2): 366–380.
[117] Sandoiu A. "Cardiovascular deaths on the rise in the US." *MedicalNewsToday* website February 2, 2019. https://www.medicalnewstoday.com/articles/324351.php

amount of exercise. It is easy to do and I can show you how.

Radiology

You will likely never meet the radiologist who makes important decisions on your care. They are a non-clinical bunch, sitting in dark rooms atop ivory towers reading medical imaging studies.

Soon, computer algorithms will replace them. Most of the studies they work on are unnecessary. Yet these elitists earn some of the highest salaries of any medical specialty.

The problems associated with radiologists, fortunately, will not directly impact you. They are a problem for the American healthcare system.

As detailed in previous sections, our medical advocacy service will help you navigate this minefield of tests that doctors will want to order. We will advise which ones to refuse and which ones to undergo.

Dentistry

I was not going to open up the can of worms found in dentistry until I saw a TV commercial that floored me. It was for a local dental chain promising same-day implants. OK. Fine. But at the end of the commercial, it stated, "Come in for a free valuation and CT-scan."

Say what? Dentists are getting in on this own-your-own-CT-scan scam like cardiologists and urgent care centers? I asked a dentist friend and he told me that this has been going on for a long time.

CT-scans for dental work are complete overkill, like hunting deer with a bazooka, and performed purely for money-making purposes. Even regular head X-rays are unnecessary as well. Never consent to this. Your head and neck have very sensitive tissue that radiation harms them more than other regions. The thyroid and pituitary glands are just two structures that are sensitive to radiation.

I never allow X-rays of my mouth, but I am not your typical patient. If you tried to decline them, your dental office would likely berate you as crazy and not even see you as a patient. However, you can easily find a dentist willing to skip the studies if you explain to them that you have read they are unnecessary and harmful.

Pediatric dentistry is where the really unscrupulous dentists thrive. There is no such thing as a pediatric dental condition that requires anything more than a basic filling (and most "cavities" found are bogus). The baby teeth are expendable. However, because CMS opened the flood gates by granting Medicaid reimbursement, horror story after horror story has been reported of child abuse at the hands of dentists.

A local TV station, WJLA-TV, produced the *Drilling for Dollars* series. CBS News also reported on the problem.[118] Multiple state and federal investigations have been performed. What they all found is indicative of routine dental practices all across the country. Evil people with dental degrees perform root canals on baby teeth, which is idiotic, among many egregious practices.

The kids are smarter than their poor uneducated parents and put up a fuss. So, a new scam as arisen. The kids are sedated in operating rooms just like a real surgery!

---

[118] "Whistleblower: Former employees take on pediatric dental chain when they suspect the company of wrongdoing." CBS News website. July 13, 2018. https://www.cbsnews.com/news/whistleblower-former-kool-smiles-employees-take-on-pediatric-dental-chain-when-they-suspect-company-of-wrongdoing/

Anesthesia is risky procedure even when trained anesthesiologists perform it, but the dentists are overseeing the process. As a result, kids have died.[119]

The routine dental procedures I just described are not just greedy scams. They should literally be categorized as criminal acts. But the dental lobbyists are very powerful. Elected prosecutors refuse to act.

---

[119] Ferguson C. "Dental board investigates a Bay Area 4-year-old's death after dentist's visit." *The Mercury Times*. May 17, 2019.

Chapter 10. What to Look for in a Healthcare Provider

By now, you are probably alarmed by American medicine. That was my intention. I aim to open eyes and stir skepticism. Far too many people blindly do whatever the doctor says, and that is not healthy.

The good news is that it is very possible to find honest and competent doctors in safe hospitals. Our medical advocacy service is not in the business of making referrals. You should make this important decision on your own. In general, these are some things to think about.

What to Look for in a Hospital

If you have been happy with the care from your existing medical system, then you should stay put. But millions of Americans are suddenly thrown into the position of needing hospital care and have little experience with the process.

Sick people do not always have the luxury of shopping around for a hospital. Try to plan in advance before an emergency arises. Ask people you know for advice. Ask yourself whether you even like your own doctor.

For any sort of surgery or elaborate test, you are better off going to a larger hospital that performs those cases more often. It has been shown in many studies that outcomes are better.

I have previously explained how so-called charity or non-profit hospitals are far too often just tax-exemption scams. But they are slightly better than publicly-traded hospitals that report to investors every three-months on earnings calls. When shareholders control the CEO of a hospital chain, very bad things happen. Doctors are pressured even more than usual to perform unnecessary care.

Ignore the irrelevant magazine rankings of "The Best Hospitals in the Country" They are marketing scams. Those struggling magazines receive payments from the medical centers. The method for ranking is arbitrary and mostly guesswork. They amount to nothing more than brand recognition rankings.

The best indicator of a good hospital for you is the staff. Choose the one where the best doctor for your need works. Quality care is all about the humans involved.

Fancy technologies rarely matter. In fact, hospitals that have spent millions purchasing the latest proton therapy or robotic surgery are often the ones where unnecessary procedures are at the greatest risk of being ordered. If a certain technology is really essential, any respectable hospital will have it.

What to Look for in a Doctor

Famous doctors are rarely the best clinicians. They have become "thought leaders" and have risen to the top for reasons unrelated to their competency as a clinical doctor. Doctors who have a hundred or more medical papers with their names on them simply demonstrate that they have gamed the academic publishing system. Trust me. One of my early surgery bosses at NYU falls into this category and is now running things at a major California university medical center.

In fact, in my experience, there tends to be an inverse relationship in surgery between the amount of papers published and the surgical competency of the doctor. Surgery residency is rigorous. The "smartest" medical students get the residency spots after they master the skills of taking multiple-choice exams that require a good memory. But then, after medical school and during residency, they have to show whether they have hand-eye coordination or can make tough real-life decisions.

In my experience, most surgeons lack the right stuff and compensate by doing time-off in the lab and publishing. Very few people have the spatial recognition and hand coordination skills required to operate. After the operation is over, few doctors know how to make decisions during crises scenarios.

When I was in surgery residency, an intern from Harvard was in the NYU surgery program, which was one of the most malignant in the country. This person would drop the fact that they went to "Harvard" early in conversations with strangers. It was a sign of insecurity because they lacked confidence in their current role as a real surgeon outside of the Harvard cocoon. Eventually, they could not handle it and quit before the year was over. They then tried her hand at Wall Street and failed there too. However, I am sure that they aced their college admission test.

Another story from residency involves a grotesquely obese heart surgery fellow. His fat fingers looked like pork sausages when crammed into rubber gloves. He was so bad that the program directors kept holding him back, not allowing him to graduate. So, he spent many years in the research lab to pad his *curriculum vitae* and matriculate. Shockingly, he ended up running the Bellevue Hospital heart surgery program. Mortality rates skyrocketed under his leadership and the state shut it down.

I have many other stories to share just like that. As I mentioned, I wrote a treatment for a potential movie or TV show. I am so sick and tired of medical dramas that glorify doctors as only competent people. There needs to be a horror film made about Hospitals. But I digress.

Back to finding a good doctor and how to go about it:

Chairs of departments often get those jobs by partnering with the drug and device industry for clinical trials. They are by no means division leaders because they are the best clinical doctors and deserve the power through meritocracy. However, there is now a trend toward hiring divisional chiefs and chairs based on the clinical prowess of the doctor. Hospitals need rainmakers who can bring in the business based on good reputations.

I mentioned previously that I played a very small role in helping Senator Grassley get the Physician Payment Sunshine Act made into law. It created a public database for doctors to report payments they receive from drug and device companies. Take the time to search your doctor.

Having stated those words of caution, most famous doctors are also good doctors. At the least, they are on top of the latest literature.

Also, do a quick Internet search of your doctor. Have they bounced around a lot? What does the hospital website bio of them state? Where did they go to medical school? Are they foreign graduates? Unlike law school, medical school is still very discriminating. To be accepted to a well-known American medical school means that the doctor does have some intelligence, usually.

"Board certification" and other accolades are essentially meaningless. Almost any doctor with a heartbeat who completes a residency program can become "board certified" Likewise, all of those framed degrees and diplomas on an office wall are the professionals' way of self-congratulating one another. They are as meaningless as the Golden Globes are to an actor. While most good doctors have these awards, so do plenty of bad doctors too.

But I still have not answered the question of how to find a good doctor. It is tough for someone who is not in the medical profession. Our medical advocacy service can help you determine this.

Hospitals that Get it Right (mostly)

Some medical centers have stellar reputations and actually deserve them. The doctors are paid and rewarded for delivering the best possible care to the patient. These shining examples have genuine cultural differences going back to the time when they were founded by a renegade doctor 100-years ago.

You have heard of some of these. Others are lesser known. Conversely, some of the most famous medical centers are frauds too. They simply spend a boatload on marketing.

Good medical centers share in common certain traits. 1) They pay the doctors with flat salaries. The doctors are not paid based on the amount of services they provide. 2) They offer bundled care options to the payers, also known as Accountable Care Organizations, or ACO's, which takes the pressure off of the bottom line. The hospitals are often part of the actual insurance company too, so there is no incentive to perform unnecessary therapies.

Most importantly, 3) the best medical centers have doctors who collaborate and communicate about individual patients. They have all of the various types of doctors and specialties under one roof acting as a caregiving team. The patient is the central hub and does not have to travel to different doctors office all over the city. Daily collaborations of the different doctors caring for a given patient occur.

The Mayo Clinic, now in several states, is one of the few medical centers that meets the criteria above and is also ranked well. Lesser known medical centers, such as Intermountain Health in Utah, Kaiser in California, and Geisinger in Pennsylvania are some other very good networks.

Sadly, almost all of the famous hospitals in coastal cities are fee-for-service programs motived to maximize cost to the payers and revenue for them. They spend a lot of money on marketing, essentially bribing magazines that create the annual "Best Hospitals" lists. Under this culture, a patient with a challenging diagnosis who would benefit from a daily meeting of multiple minds is instead seen by doctors working in silos. Notes written in the electronic medical records are the extent of "communication" Patients are shuffled all over the city for various appointments. The care provided is far from optimal.

Since the vast majority of American hospitals are structured in the wrong ways, creating perverse incentives not aligned with the best interest of the patient, our medical advocacy service helps you get the best possible healthcare from these providers. Even under suboptimal conditions, it is possible to receive safe and effective care. But you need a smart advocate.

Chapter 11. How to Protect Yourself

I have certainly alarmed you by now about how the American healthcare system really works, how can you protect yourself and get the most out of your healthcare provider? Obviously, I recommend using our medical advocacy service. But if you are not currently ill and would rather wait, then the following tips can help you prepare.

Have Family Members by Your Bedside

The most important asset you can have to prevent adverse outcomes is a strong support network of friends and family. Ideally, one of them would be a nurse or doctor. Your inner circle are the best medical advocates. Our service can just augment them.

There is no certification or degree required to be a medical advocate. As the population ages and demand for advocates grows, I predict that there will soon be an industry of regular folks becoming advocates. Obviously, medical experience does not hurt.

Most hospitals now have single-occupant rooms with chairs that can be turned into beds for a visitor. There is nothing wrong with a family member staying by the bedside for much of the day.

If someone is in the room with you, they act as a scarecrow to keep the bad actors away. A constant presence sends a strong message to the nurses and doctors. You will be treated more like a V.I.P. if they see that others care about you. Our advocacy service can provide nurses to sit by the bedside and monitor the hospital nursing care.

But most people are not that fortunate. Their spouse has died or their children are not close at hand. What can you do then?

In the ER

Your first encounter with the hospital will likely be in the emergency room. The ER is a miserable and intimidating place. The staff know it and act differently than in other settings. Pleasantries, such as a proper introduction, are often skipped. The ER staff can be quite rude, to put it mildly (try to go to a good outpatient urgent care center instead).

It is very important that you know your legal rights in the ER, if you are fortunate enough to be alert and oriented. If you have a family member helping you in the ER, they can be your voice.

The first thing you need to know in the ER is whom is your doctor in charge of your care. In teaching hospitals, medical students or residents will see you after the triage nurses. They all have white coats and look like doctors, but there is an "attending" doctor in charge who will make any final decisions. Find out whom that is.

If you ask someone in a white coat, "Are you my doctor?", and they reply with a dodgy answer, such as, "I am taking care of you.", they are likely not a medical doctor, but rather a nurse practitioner. In an effort to meet the overwhelming patient volume seen in many urban hospitals, states have passed laws giving nurse practitioners the same powers as a medical doctor. The problem is that they have far less training than a medical doctor.

Either your support team or you should have a small notebook in which you write down the names of everyone treating you. The notebook is a good excuse to ask everyone to state their name and job title.

The ER is where many of the diagnostic tests will be performed. Be sure to ask what labs and medical imaging tests have been ordered. More importantly, ask why? I have previously explained how many of the most common tests are unnecessary.

Do Not Sign Contracts Without Reading Them

When you step foot into a hospital, you will be barraged with multiple lengthy legal forms, which are binding contracts. Even under ideal settings, when you are healthy and alert, you are not a lawyer and are incapable of understanding them. It is disgraceful how hospitals take advantage of the vulnerable patients with no options and require them to sign away rights.

The bottom line is this: never sign a contract if you are not clear what it is. You will need to sign a contract granting your consent for treatment, as well as forms that detail your insurance and other information. But the contracts they want you to sign that indemnify the hospital, or claim that you are aware of and agree to the terms of the lengthy mystery document, are not forms you need to sign on the spot with a hospital employee looking over your shoulder.

When you are recovering and getting ready to leave the hospital, this is when the "case managers" start to come into the room and tell you to sign away your life. The forms essentially have you agreeing that you authorized everything they ever did to you. They are unconscionable contracts.

Whenever a contract is presented to you, in any setting, tell the counter party that you want to read it carefully and get back with them. If they pressure you, then that is a red flag.

The vast majority of patients never stand up for their rights and sign anything given to them. The hospital employee will likely pressure you to sign. Tell them to back off. However, this is easier said than done, and why our medical advocacy services are of use.

Questions to Ask When Admitted to the Hospital

Once you are admitted to the hospital and placed into a room on some high floor in a medical tower, what should you do then? The process is similar to the ER.

Use your same notebook and track the names of everyone walking into the room. Most hospitals now have white-boards in the room that list the names of the nurses on duty, etc. However, the identity of the actual doctor accountable for your care is often unknown. Be sure to ask, "Who is the admitting doctor in charge?"

When hospital staff see a patient or their family taking notes, they take notice and treat you with more respect. Do not be afraid to ask basic questions.

Proactively Inform Your Normal Doctors

As I explained previously, few American medical centers are as good as the Mayo Clinic at having a true team oversee your care and communicate daily. This used to be the main function of your family doctor, but no longer. Your primary care doctor will not likely visit you in the hospital. They usually are not even notified.

You need to take it upon yourself to tell your normal crew of medical caregivers what is going on. Call your primary care doctor and tell them that you have been admitted to the hospital. Ask them to look at the latest tests and explain the results. Ask them if they agree with the decisions being made.

Checklist to Reduce the Chances of Harm

Prior to Becoming Sick

- o Do your homework. Find the best doctors and hospitals.
- o Identify friends and family willing to be with you if you need to go to the hospital.
- o Have a discussion with them. Do not assume they will show up and support you.
- o Designate a primary advocate to whom the others will report. This helps avoid chaos once you become ill. Squabbling family members and egos are a big problem once you become sick.
- o Discuss a living will, which specifies how you want to be cared for when you are unable to make the decisions yourself.
- o Buy this book.

In the Emergency Room

- o Try to gather your advocacy network, if you are able.
- o Buy this book and bring it with you.
- o Collect names of people treating you.
- o Specifically ask for the training and titles of caregivers.
- o Always ask whether a medical imaging study is essential. Tell the doctor that you have read how CT-scans, etc. are often unnecessary.
- o Notify your family doctor.

Once You Are Admitted to the Hospital

- o Identify the doctor in charge of your care.
- o Have your advocacy team spend time in your hospital room.
- o Collect names of all caregivers.
- o Try to sit up and walk if you are safely able to do so.
- o Politely question the need for all medical imaging studies and procedures—make the doctor explain the rationale.
- o When case managers or nurses ask you to sign a contract (i.e. any piece of paper), tell them that you need to read it and set it aside—do not be pressured into signing anything on the spot.

Prior to Going Home

- o If you do not feel safe going home, due to lack of supportive care, refuse to be discharged until a proper acute-care outpatient facility is found.
- o If you feel that you are being rushed out of the hospital too soon, escalate the matter with the hospital administrator and the doctor in charge of your care.

Once the Bills Arrive

- o Never pay any bills from the hospital until you verify that they are not scams.
- o Have your insurance company verify that the bills are legitimate.
- o Speak to a service that provides help understanding complex bills.

Chapter 12. What is the Medical Advocate Service?

What exactly is this medical advocacy service we offer? In the foreword, I explained how the idea arose after acting as an advocate for my parents. I have also tried to explain how your family and/or you can act as your own advocate.

The checklist that I provided above is easier said than done. Our services can assist with the process.

Hospitals and people in white coats are extremely intimidating. Very few people feel comfortable even asking for the names of the caregivers, much less challenging an unconscionable contract pushed into their faces to "sign...or else" Our service does this for you.

We also provide nurses to sit by the bedside to monitor the care and make sure that proper protocol is followed. Plenty of reputable hospitals still allow bad nursing care to happen, resulting in bed sores or worse. Many caregivers do not wash their hands, despite this being preached to them. The dosages of drugs administered are often wrong. Some staff can be flagrantly abusive to elderly.

We then act as the liaison between all of your caregivers. It is sad, actually, that we can even be of added benefit here because this used to be the main function of your primary care doctor. With our help, the doctors are all on the same page. Test results are seen within hours, not days.

Throughout the process, we act as your second-opinion too. Because we are not biased by financial conflicts of interest that favor the caregivers, our opinions will not steer you toward treatments that you do not need.

When it comes time for your discharge, we make sure that you are not forced to sign unconscionable contracts. You are not legally obligated to sign any discharge paper. You can walk out of a hospital at any time you like, if you are mentally competent.

We also advocate for your rights when "case managers" try to intimidate you into leaving the hospital too soon. Because hospitals are paid flat rates per a diagnosis, the shorter you stay, the more profit they make. Case managers have quotas and mandates to kick people out as soon as possible.

In many cases, patients are well enough to leave the hospital, but lack the support structure in their homes to go straight home. Finding a facility that handles these in-between stages is fraught with problems. The hospital social workers often do not do an adequate job. They refer to facilities that are within their medical center network, keeping the revenue in-house. We help select the best rehabilitation hospitals, regardless of networks, and then follow up with you there at those facilities.

If you need a long-term nursing home, we can assist by preventing abuse and neglect. As I mentioned previously, nursing homes are far less regulated than hospitals and bad things occur on a daily basis. However, if the patient has family support and a good advocate, the care delivered is much better.

I know the nursing home setting far better than almost any other type of doctor. As I mentioned, I have treated patients with chronic wounds in these facilities. Twenty-years ago, I pioneered the entire concept of doctors visiting nursing homes to treat wounds.

Of note, we do not actually replace your doctors or act as a doctor treating you. Medical advocacy is an advisory service.

After you receive medical or surgical care, the bills start to come in. I explained previously how most medical centers are losing money. These financial pressures are leading to unethical billing practices. We assist you with challenging those surprise bills and fighting scams.

The cost for our medical advocacy service often pays for itself. However, the peace of mind cannot be measured in dollars.

If you are interested in learning more, please call us and we will have more thorough discussion. Our contact information is:

The Quality of Life Clinic
http://qolhospitals.com/
(212) 945-7252
Steve@QOLclinic.com

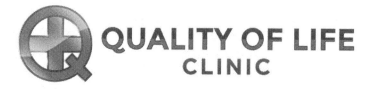

Acknowledgements

I have to give a ton of credit to Christopher Attinger, MD for the term "medical advocate" and this book. In early 2019, as he and I worked on a project to create a new paradigm for treating chronic wounds, I was telling him about my experiences with my parents. He mentioned how crucial it is to have a "medical advocate" Months later, as I was driving from Ohio to Florida, I had the idea to start this service for others.

Dr. Attinger is a rare doctor these days. He is a dedicated surgeon who salvages legs, preventing amputations. He is a Vietnam War purple heart recipient, Harvard-trained surgeon, and NYU-trained plastic surgeon. Working out of Georgetown Hospital, he has been one of the most respected wound care doctors in the world for many decades. He sees the sickest of the sick patients. Dr. Attinger knows that those patients with medical advocates fare much better.

Peter Pronovost, MD, PhD, has also been a big help. He is one of the leading experts on the topics of medical errors and improving patient care. The Sectary of Health and Human Services recently appointed him as the chairman of the Quality Summit.[120] He pioneered the safety checklist concept while at Johns Hopkins.

Numerous other people deserve credit for supporting my idea when I explained it to them as well. The responses have been uniformly positive and gave me the confidence to go ahead and write this book.

---

[120] "HHS Announces Quality Summit to Streamline and Improve Quality Programs across Government" U.S. Department of Health and Human Services. July 9, 2019.

And finally, last but not least, my parents deserve credit. Interactions I had with their caregivers in 2018 and 2019 are what directly led to this book and advocacy service.

Steven E. Greer, MD: Curriculum Vitae

Education

- **M.D.**: The Ohio State University College of Medicine, Columbus, Ohio
- **B.A.**: The Ohio State University Fisher College of Business. Major: Finance:

Medical Work Experience

- 2013-current: **Quality of Life Clinic** Founder/CEO. Concierge medicine, wound care/limb salvage, and medical advocacy services
- 1998-2000: **Research Project Director**- New York Veterans Affairs Medical Center/ The Institute of Reconstructive Plastic Surgery, New York University Medical Center. Responsible for the operations of a two-year $408,000 multicenter wound healing research project and management of a Ph.D. Research Nurse (see Grants section).
- 1998-2000: **Postdoctoral Clinical Wound Healing Fellow**- The Developmental Biology and Repair Laboratory of Michael T. Longakcr, The Institute of Reconstructive Plastic Surgery, New York University Medical Center
- 1997-2000: **General Surgery/Plastic Surgery Residency**- New York University Medical Center
- 1996-1997: **General Surgery-** Mount Sinai Hospital and Jackson Memorial Hospital, Miami

Academic Projects

- 1998-2000: **The Bellevue Wound Healing and Research Center**: initiated the creation of a multidisciplinary wound healing and research center.
- 1998-2000: **The New York University Wound Healing Center**: after the Bellevue wound center, was invited by the Chairman of Plastic Surgery to help develop the NYU wound healing center.

Financial Work Experience

- 2007-current: **The Healthcare Channel** (http://thehcc.tv/) Founder/CEO. Provides business information in multimedia format to institutional investors and healthcare executives via subscription.
- 2007-2011: **Fox Business Network** and **Wall Street Journal** contributor. Contract partner with **Thomson Reuters** for healthcare content creation.
- 2005-2006: **Merrill Lynch** Strategic Investment Group. Director. Global Healthcare Portfolio Manager for a $10B long/short internal hedge fund
- 2002-2005: **The SG Healthcare Fund**. Founder
- 2001-2002: **Sigma Capital** Management. Partner. A subsidiary fund of SAC Capital
- 2000-2001: **Donaldson, Lufkin & Jenrette** Securities Corporation, then **Credit-Suisse First Boston** after the merger with DLJ. Research Analyst, Medical Device/Diagnostics/Biotech

Academic Research and Publications

Books and Mainstream Publications

1. Greer SE. **"The Medical Advocate"** New York. Quality of Life Clinic publishing. 2019
2. Greer SE (Editor-in-Chief), Benhaim P, Lorenz HP, Chang J, Hedrick MH (Eds.). **"The Handbook of Plastic Surgery"** New York: Marcel Dekker, 2004
3. Greer SE. **"Inside ObamaCare's Grant-Making"** Op-Ed in The Wall Street Journal. June 4, 2012
4. Greer SE. **"Pork is Clogging CMMI's Arteries"** Letter section in The Wall Street Journal. June 20, 2012

Grants

1. B2108RC/VA Merit Review Grant, 10/01/99-10/01/2001 (Principal Investigator: Longaker)[121] awarded $408,280: **Investigation of Subatmospheric Pressure Dressing on Pressure Ulcer Healing.**
2. NCRR M01 RR00096, 6/21/99-6/20/2000 (Principal Investigator: Longaker) **Controlled Study of Subatmospheric Pressure Dressing on Below-Knee Amputation Wounds.** The NIH-funded General Clinical Research Center, physically located at Bellevue but a distinct entity, accepted the application for the study listed above to be conducted at their facility. (The VA also approved this grant, but did not provide funding given that they had funded the other study)

---

[121] Steven Greer designed the trials, wrote the grant applications, and conducted all clinical care and data gathering. However, being a resident in training lacking "attending" status, Michael Longaker was listed as PI

3. NCRR M01 RR00096, 6/21/99-6/20/2000 (Principal Investigator: Greer): **Application of Outcome Data to Pressure Ulcer Healing.** The NIH-funded General Clinical Research Center, physically located at Bellevue Hospital but a distinct entity, accepted the application for the study listed above to be conducted at their facility.
4. Private Industry Grant, KCI inc., 10/31/98-10/31/99 (Principal Investigator: Greer) $64,000, 1998: **A Controlled Study Comparing the Effectiveness of Subatmospheric Pressure Dressing to Normal Saline Wet-To-Moist Dressing on Pressure Ulcers**

Journal Articles

1. Greer SE, Matarasso A, Wallach S, Simon G, Longaker MT: **The Importance of the Nasal-to-Cervical Relationship to the Profile and Rhinoplasty Surgery.** *Plastic and Reconstructive Surgery.* 108(2):522-31; discussion 532-5. 2001
2. Greer SE, Grossi EA, Chin D, Longaker MT. **Subatmospheric Pressure Dressing for Closure of Saphenous Vein Donor-Site Wound Complications.** *Annals of Thoracic Surgery*, 71(3):1038-1040, 2001
3. Greer SE: **A Lesson from the High-Tech Economic Boom: Utilize the Competitive Advantage of Plastic Surgery.** *Plastic and Reconstructive Surgery*, 107(2):598-601, 2001
4. Puckett CL, Greer SE: **A Lesson from the High-Tech Economic Boom: Utilize the Competitive Advantage of Plastic Surgery.** Discussion. *Plastic and Reconstructive Surgery*, 107(2):602-603, 2001
5. Greer SE: **Whither Subatmospheric Pressure Dressing?** Editorial. *Ann Plast Surg*, 45(3):332-4, 2000

6. Greer SE, Matarasso A, Wallach S, Simon G, Longaker MT: **The Nasal-to-Cervical Relationship of Rhinoplasty Surgery.** *Plastic Surgical Forum*, 2000

7. Greer SE, Longaker MT, Cutting C, McCarthy JG, Shaw W, Lorenz HP: **The Gold Standard for Acceptable Resolution of Projected Digital Photographic Images in Plastic Surgery.** *Plastic Surgical Forum,* 2000

8. Greer SE, MD, Adelman M, MD, Kasabian A, MD, Galiano R, MD, Scott R, MD, Longaker MT, MD: **The Use of Subatmospheric Pressure Dressing to Close Lymphocutaneous Fistulas of the Groin.** *Brit J Plast Surg*, 53(6):484-487, 2000

9. Matarasso A, Greer SE, Longaker MT: **The True Hanging Columella: Simplified Diagnosis and Treatment Using a Modified Direct Approach.** *Plastic and Reconstructive Surgery*, 106(2):469-474, 2000

10. Matarasso A, Greer SE, Longaker MT: **The True Hanging Columella: Simplified Diagnosis and Treatment Using a Modified Direct Approach.** *Plastic Surgical Forum*, 2000

11. Greer SE, Longaker MT, Margiotta M: **Preliminary Results from a Multicenter, Randomized, Controlled, Study of the Use of Subatmospheric Pressure Dressing for Pressure Ulcer Healing.** *Wound Repair and Regeneration.* 7(4); 255, 1999

12. Greer SE, Longaker MT, Margiotta M, Mathews AJ, Kasabian A: **The Use of Subatmospheric Pressure Dressing for the Coverage of Radial Forearm Free Flap Donor-Site Exposed Tendon Complications.** *Ann Plast Surg.* 43(5):551-554, November 1999

13. Greer SE, Duthie E, Cartolano B, Koehler KM, Maydick-Youngberg D, Longaker MT: **Techniques for Applying Subatmospheric Pressure Dressing to Wounds in Difficult Regions of Anatomy.** *Journal of Wound Ostomy Continence Nursing.* 26(5); 250-3, September 1999

14. Greer SE, Kasabian A, Thorne C, Borud L, Sims CD, Hsu M: **The Use of a Subatmospheric Pressure Dressing to Salvage a Gustilo Grade IIIB Open Tibia Fracture with Concomitant Osteomyelitis and Avert a Free Flap.** Letter. *Annals of Plastic Surgery,* 41(6); 687, Dec 1998

Presentations and Television Appearances

1. Greer SE, Regular guest on **The Fox Business Network**, 2008 to 2013
2. Greer SE, Guest on **CNBC's Larry Kudlow Show**, 2013
3. Greer SE, Guest on **MSNBC's Dylan Ratigan Show**, 2012
4. Greer SE, FDA **Rejection of Cyberonics Depression Device**. Kudlow and Cramer Show. CNBC. August 12, 2004
5. Greer SE, Guest on **CNBC's Kudlow and Cramer Show**. CNBC. April 27, 2004
6. Matarasso, A, Greer SE, Wallach S, Longaker MT, Simon, G. **The Importance of the Nasal-to-Cervical Relationship in Rhinoplasty Surgery**. American Association of Plastic Surgeons-80th Annual Meeting. Charleston, SC. May 16, 2001.

7. Greer SE, Longaker MT, Cutting C, McCarthy JG, Shaw W, Lorenz HP: **The Gold Standard for Acceptable Resolution of Projected Digital Photographic Images in Plastic Surgery.** American Society of Plastic Surgeons- 69th annual meeting, Los Angeles, California, October 15, 2000

8. Matarasso A, Greer SE, Longaker MT: **The True Hanging Columella: Simplified Diagnosis and Treatment Using a Modified Direct Approach.** American Society of Plastic Surgeons- 69th annual meeting, Los Angeles, California, October 15, 2000

9. Greer SE, Matarasso A, Wallach S, Simon G, Longaker MT: **The Nasal-to-Cervical Relationship of Rhinoplasty Surgery.** Accepted for poster presentation at the 69th annual ASPS meeting, Los Angeles, California, October 15, 2000

10. Matarasso A, Greer SE, Longaker MT: **The True Hanging Columella: Simplified Diagnosis and Treatment Using a Modified Direct Approach.** Presented at the fifth annual Rhinoplasty Society meeting, Orlando, Florida, May 11, 2000

11. Greer SE, Matarasso A, Wallach S, Simon G, Longaker MT: **The Nasal-to-Cervical Relationship of Rhinoplasty Surgery.** Presented at the fifth annual Rhinoplasty Society meeting, Orlando, Florida, May 2000

12. Greer SE, Houston V: **A Proposal to Treat Land Mine Amputation Wounds Using Subatmospheric Pressure Dressing.** Presented at the World Health Organization, 2 United Nations Plaza, New York, NY to the Executive Director of the WHO, Dr. Bassani, November 18, 1999

13. Greer SE, Longaker MT, Margiotta M, Mathews AJ, Kasabian A: **The Use of Subatmospheric Pressure Dressing for the Coverage of Radial Forearm Free Flap Donor-Site Exposed Tendon Complications.**

Presented at the International Society of Reconstructive Microsurgeons, UCLA Medical Center, Los Angeles, CA June 22, 1999

14. Greer SE: **Subatmospheric Pressure Dressing: Clinical Applications and Research Opportunities.** Presented at the Grand Rounds for the Division of Plastic Surgery, Yale University, New Haven, CT, April 15, 1999

15. Greer SE, Longaker MT, Margiotta M: **Preliminary Results from a Multicenter, Randomized, Controlled, Study of the Use of Subatmospheric Pressure Dressing for Pressure Ulcer Healing.** Accepted for presentation at the Joint Meeting of the European Tissue Repair Society and The Wound Healing Society. Bordeaux, France August, 1999

16. Greer SE: **Subatmospheric Pressure Dressing: Orthopedic Clinical Applications and Research Opportunities.** Jacoby Hospital Orthopedic Conference. New York, NY January, 1999

17. Clarkson MW, Greer SE, Sullivan MJ, Danahey D, Siegle RJ,: **The Effects Of Estrogen on Photoaged Skin and Chemical Peeling**. Presented at the 1994 William H. Saunders Lectureship, Columbus, Ohio.

18. Greer SE, Townsend M: **Motorcycle Helmet Use and Mechanisms of Injury**. Landacre Research Conference. Columbus, Ohio, 1993

Testimonials

"This is a sobering and compelling book that explains why your health and well-being are usually not the primary concern when you enter your health care system as a patient. Competing interests of healthcare bureaucracy, procedure-driven interventions, pharmaceuticals, regulations, etc. all muddy the waters.

The book is fascinating reading and a must for those both in healthcare as well as anyone who is, or has family that is about to be, hospitalized. It points out the potential pitfalls for patients and their families. Staying informed and having access to an advocate will increase the chances for receiving appropriate care."

Chris Attinger, MD
Professor, Director of the Center for Wound Healing
Plastic & Reconstructive Surgery
MedStar Georgetown University Hospital

"As the American system of health care moves farther and farther away from a patient-focused model, a book like this is invaluable for the average consumer of medical care to learn how to make their way through this system without a professional advocate. Dr. Greer's book helps to bridge the growing gap in the doctor-patient relationship"

Lawrence Brecht, DDS
Department of Plastic Surgery
New York University Medical Center

"Impressive. Well done. This is an important book.

You could be the most impactful investigative journalist, as well as investor and innovator."

Peter Pronovost, MD, PhD
University Hospitals, Cleveland
Chair of the "Quality Committee" for The HHS
Former Professor, Johns Hopkins
Former Chief Medical Officer, UnitedHealthcare
MacArthur Genius Award winner as pioneer of hospital safety checklists

---

"This is VERY interesting. I like being part of your book too. . . A little notoriety 😊 😁. It truly is a Great Read.

I am so happy and Proud to be the mom of such a gifted writer and author. You would make your Grandma Reid very proud too. She was a high school English teacher and good writer (and speaker) herself. Her genetics were passed on down to YOU and me."

Martha Greer
My Mother

Index

Attention Deficit and
Hyperactivity Disorder,
65
Attention-
deficit/hyperactivity
disorder, 50
Atul Gawande, 87
Avastin, 76
azisothymidine, 30
azithromycin, 64
AZT, 30

B

bankruptcy, 12, 13, 14, 15
bennies, 51
Bernie Sanders, 27
Big Tobacco, 34
black-box, 49
Boehringer Ingelheim
Pharmaceuticals, 70
Boston Scientific, 55
BRCA gene mutations,
120
Bristol-Meyers Squibb,
70
Bristol-Myers Squibb, 54
Byetta, 46

C

C. diff, 65
CABG, 98, 100
Caffeine, 66
cane sugar, 36

cardiology mafia, 80
Cardiopulmonary
Resuscitation, 101
Carotid artery
ultrasonography, 92
carotid endarterectomy,
92
case managers, vii, 140
Cathryn Jakobson Ramin,
97
Centers for Medicare and
Medicaid Services, 10,
24, 26, 41
Centers for Medicare and
Medicaid Services
(CMS), 10, 24, 26, 41
Clostridium difficile, 64
CMS, 10, 21, 24, 26, 41
Computed tomography
pulmonary
angiography, 92
contracts, 140
Convatec, 54
coronary artery bypass,
94
coronary artery bypass
graft surgery, 100
coronary calcium
screening, 99
coronary stenting, 92
cortisol, 68
Coumadin, 70
CPR, 101

flora, 64
fluoxetine, 49
fluvoxamine, 50

G

gatekeepers, 83
Geisinger, 135
Gertrude Elion, 30
ghrelin, 37
GI bleed, iii, v
GlaxoSmithKline, 30, 53
GLP-1 agonists, 46
gonorrhea, 32
Great Depression, 25
Guidant, 79

H

H&Ps, 116
Harmful Food, 35
Harvard, 12, 13, 14, 18, 30, 52, 87
Health and Human Services, 18, 24
Health Insurance Portability and Accountability Act, 112
Health Insurance Portability and Accountability Act of 1996, 112
Healthcare Channel, 63

heart attack, 16, 46, 60, 95, 98, 126
HHS, 24
high-fructose corn syrup, 36
Himmelstein, 12, 13, 14, 15
hip replacement, 96
history and physicals, 116
Hitler, 52
HIV, 30
Holmesburg Prison, 32
Horizant, 53
hormone replacement therapy, 73
hospitalists, 106
Howard Schaeffer, 30
HRT, 73
Humira, 69, 76
hydrochlorothiazide, 64
hydrocodone/acetaminophen, 57
hyperlipidemia, 46
Hypertension, 126
hypovolemic shock, 101

I

ICD, 79
ICU, 22, 101
Immunotherapy, 30
impaired glucose metabolism, 45

Implantable cardioverter
    defibrillators, 79
in vitro diagnostics, 94
Institute of Medicine, 40,
    84
insulin, 37, 45
Intermountain Health,
    135

J

Jackson Memorial
    Hospital, vi
Januvia, 46
John F. Kennedy, 26
John Glenn, 80
Johnny Cash, 51
Johnson & Johnson, 55,
    70, 79
Jonas Salk, 30
JPMorgan, 27
JUPITER, 60

K

Kaiser, 15, 135
kickbacks, 55, 83
knee implants, 79
Knee scoping, 96

L

legal forms, 140
legal rights, 138
Leonardo da Vinci, 29

Lipitor, 46, 60, 62, 76,
    125
lisinopril, 64
Louis Pasteur, 29
Luvox, 50
Lyndon B. Johnson, 26

M

major depressive
    disorders, 49
malaria, 32
mammograms, 93
Mammograms, 93
Martin Shkreli, 77
Mayo Clinic, 88, 135
medical device lobbyists,
    79
Medical Errors, 84
medicalizing, 45
Medicare-for-all, 12
Medicines and Healthcare
    products Regulatory
    Agency, 49
Medtronic, 55
Merrill Lynch, 55
methylphenidate, 51
Modern surgery, 29
Mount Carmel, 87

N

National Academies of
    Science, 40

National Healthcare
Expenditure, 10, 76
Nazis, 31
Neil Armstrong, 100
Neulasta, 122
Neupogen, 122
NNT, 56
Nobel Prize, 30
Norvasc, 64
Number Needed to Treat,
56
Nuremberg Code, 32
nurse practitioner, 138
NYU Stern School of
Business, 54

O

Obamacare, 17, 21, 24,
27, 82, 110, 111
Onglyza, 46
open-heart surgery, 30,
80, 100
Opioids Pain Pills, 57
Oprah Winfrey, 124
out-of-pocket costs, 12,
17, 121
oxycodone, 57
Oxycontin, 57

P

papillary thyroid, 120
Pediatric dentistry, 128
Peter Pronovost, 86

Peter Safar, 101
Physician Payments
Sunshine Act, 82
pituitary apoplexy, iv
Poisoner in Chief, 33
Pradaxa, 70
Praluent, 62
Prediabetes, 45
premature ventricular
contraction, 66
preventricular
contractions, 67
Prinivil, 64
Prostate cancer, 120
Psychiatric Drugs, 35
PVC, 67

R

Regeneron, 62
Repatha, 62
restenosis, 98
Ritalin, 51
rivaroxoban, 70
Robert Lustig, MD, 36
rosuvastatin, 60

S

Sackler, 58
Sanford Bernstein, 79
Sanofi, 62
second-opinions, 88, 89
sepsis, 101

violence, 107

W

Warren, 13, 14, 27
Warren Buffet, 27
Wellcome, 30
whistleblowers, 82
WHO, 40
Wilhelm Conrad
  Röntgen, 29
William Boden, MD, 81
William Halsted, MD, 29
William Husel, 87
William Maisel, 80

William T. G. Morton, 29
WJLA-TV, 128
World Health
  Organization, 40

X

Xarelto, 70
XenoPort, 53

Z

Zestril, 64
Zithromax, 64
Zocor, 60
Z-pack, 64

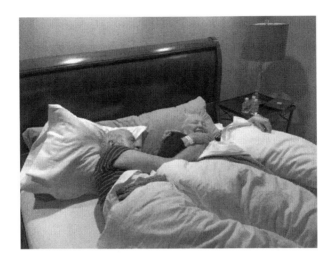

My mother sleeping without pain for the first time after her pituitary apoplexy episode, next to my father. This was the first night after leaving the hospital. She still has the hospital bracelet on. It was so disturbing to see her in agonizing pain in the hospital, only able to sleep while medicated.